I need to thank all of the people who have given their support, but I want to give a special thanks to Brigit and Lynne, without whom I would undoubtedly have given up.

I dedicate this book to my Father.

When the world was a dark place and I was lost, he appeared and suggested a path.

I finally realised, that in every dark time, he was there.

What greater gift can a father give to a son?

Contents

~O~

ANY COMMERCIAL USE OR PUBLICATION OF ALL
OR PART OF DOCUMENTS ON THIS SITE IS STRICTLY
PROHIBITED, WITHOUT PRIOR WRITTEN
AUTHORISATION FROM:

WWW.MONKEYONMYSHOULDER.CO.UK.
(MONKEY@MONKEYONMYSHOULDER.CO.UK)

THE COPYRIGHT REMAINS WITH THE AUTHOR
UNDER ALL CONDITIONS.

THIS DOCUMENT IS PROVIDED "AS IS," AND
COPYRIGHT HOLDERS MAKE NO
REPRESENTATIONS OR WARRANTIES, EXPRESS OR
IMPLIED, INCLUDING, BUT NOT LIMITED TO,
WARRANTIES OF MERCHANTABILITY, FITNESS FOR
A PARTICULAR PURPOSE, NON-INFRINGEMENT, OR
TITLE; THAT THE CONTENTS OF THE DOCUMENT
ARE SUITABLE FOR ANY PURPOSE; NOR THAT THE
IMPLEMENTATION OF SUCH CONTENTS WILL NOT
INFRINGE ANY THIRD PARTY PATENTS,
COPYRIGHTS, TRADEMARKS OR OTHER RIGHTS.

COPYRIGHT HOLDERS WILL NOT BE LIABLE FOR
ANY DIRECT, INDIRECT, SPECIAL OR
CONSEQUENTIAL DAMAGES ARISING OUT OF ANY
USE OF THE DOCUMENT OR THE PERFORMANCE OR
IMPLEMENTATION OF THE CONTENTS THEREOF.

Introduction

You are probably reading this book because either you or a loved one has a drink problem. Life has reached the stage where you need an answer, but the answers seem frightening.

Alcoholism is an illness and Alcoholics Anonymous has meetings and a "program" to help people recover from it. Whilst the very name Alcoholics Anonymous seems shrouded in mystery, there isn't anything suspicious or veiled about them. At every meeting, they start by reading out the "pre-amble" the complete explanation of what AA is:

> *ALCOHOLICS ANONYMOUS is a fellowship of men and women who share their experience, strength and hope with each other that they may solve their common problem and help others to recover from alcoholism. The only requirement for membership is a desire to stop drinking. There are no dues or fees for A.A. membership; we are self-supporting through our own contributions. A.A. is not allied with any sect, denomination, politics, organization or institution; does not wish to engage in any controversy; neither endorses nor opposes any causes. Our primary purpose is to stay sober and help other alcoholics to achieve sobriety.*
>
> *(Reprinted with permission of The A.A. Grapevine, Inc.)*

The statement: The only requirement for membership is a desire to stop drinking is the first hurdle. If we knew how to stop, we wouldn't need help and we often scream out - HOW?   Our answer is in the acronym, providing we can achieve three conditions - Honest, Open Minded, Willing, we can recover:

Honest, when we have a drink problem, we feel exposed and unwilling to acknowledge the full depth of our problems (even to ourselves).

Open minded, some of what we will encounter will seem alien to us and this can cause us to reject an idea before we have fully appreciated its relevance.

Willing, rather than allowing ourselves to be crippled by secrecy or a closed mind we need to be able to say – "Ok, I give up, tell me how to do it and I will try my best".

If this is the first time that you have looked for help, you are almost certainly unhappy with the way your life has unfolded. Isolated, you see others are enjoying life, but you don't seem to be able to join them. You are not alone in this feeling. In fact, we have all felt this way. Drinking is certainly a part of your life and somebody might have suggested it could be getting out of hand. You may not agree, but you are now at the stage where you are willing to look for a solution.

If you have been trying to work through the AA program for some time you have probably been going to meetings and have managed to stop drinking. You have looked at the program and don't understand it. Because you have been around for a while, you are scared to ask what you think are basic questions, because people will laugh at your lack of knowledge. Although you don't know it, you are not alone and we have all felt like this as well.

Please allow me to introduce…

…Myself.

I am just a bloke who got in a mess with booze. I arrived at the doors of AA without a hope in the world and found a worthwhile life. I don't claim to be anything special, but I do have a good memory. As part of my own recovery, I have discussed the program with many people and I am certain that there is only one obstacle – our own thinking. It is a cycle. We struggle, we become willing to acknowledge our problem, we honestly discuss it and when we are open to learn, a light suddenly comes on. We look back and cannot believe how we made our recovery so difficult.

I have compiled the "light bulb" moments and common pitfalls I have encountered over the years to pass on to other people.

AA does not currently endorse this book, but I hope you find that it contains helpful ideas and suggestions if you try to adopt the program into your life.

…The Monkey!

The illness is "awoken" when I drink and a symptom of the illness is that I have a compulsion to drink more. It can actually feel like the illness has a voice and intelligence and is trying to manipulate me into taking a drink.

I have an image of my illness as a monkey. Not a cute little fur ball of fun, but a devious, clever and tenacious monkey (who happens to talk as well). This image came to me when I used to get home, open the door and "wham" a feeling of dread and hopelessness would drop from the door jamb and land on the back of my neck. It was an empty home and as I entered, feelings of despair and darkness seemed to wreath about me. In this emptiness, whispered thoughts crept into my mind, "you won't make it through the night". It was too much to bear. Within seconds, I changed from happy and safe into lonely and scared. Clearly, there was an invisible talking monkey waiting to drop on my shoulder when I got home.

A more clinical view would be that I have an addiction that triggers a subconscious craving, but I find it easier to imagine the image of a monkey trying to trick me into feeding it.

Here are some of the ways the monkey messes up our lives:

It whispers constantly "Go on, nobody will know, you deserve a long cool drink after the day you had…" or "Take a drink. That will teach them to treat you this way…"

It covers our eyes to stop us seeing what is really happening. At a party, it can turn a troll into the most attractive person in the room and we end up in a relationship that is doomed to fail.

It covers our ears, we become deaf to the pleas of our families and we won't listen when we get our final warnings from jobs.

That is the monkey, it constantly whispers insinuations, it schemes and swings around our heads covering our eyes and ears. Where did the monkey come from and how did we acquire such a spiteful companion?

For some of us it first shows up when we hit a low patch. We are sitting feeling sorry for ourselves and it wanders up and seems to be helping us through our problems. For others who feel restrained and shy, it arrives with the promise of confidence. For those who already enjoy the bright lights, it promises even brighter lights.

Through promises or by stealth it becomes a part of our life. We become fond of our new friend and ask it to move in. The guest settles down and makes its home within us. It rides on our shoulder whispering new ways to enjoy life, sometimes it pushes a bit too far, but as with any good friend, we forgive and make up. As time passes, the whisperings become darker and it no longer has to provide the gifts it once did. It can demand whatever it wants and we are now unable to evict it.

…how to use this book

It is a guidebook. A good guidebook offers simple suggestions and guidance to you as you visit a new place. It suggests places to go and a good way to get there. It explains basic problems you may encounter such as taxis, local holidays and customs.

We don't normally read a travel guide from cover to cover with the same intensity we would read a novel. We normally use it in three ways:

- Beforehand we flip through the pages and make a plan of what we are going to do during our trip.

- Whilst we travel, we use the maps and tour suggestions as a guide.

- When we are in trouble, we flick through the pages remembering that we saw a page of surgery opening hours somewhere near the back.

I suggest that you try to use this book in the same way.

The book is deliberately broken into three sections:

Getting Started- I suggest you read this section before embarking. It is only short and I hope that it will cover the essentials for the journey.

The Program- This section is a practical guide towards doing each step. It focuses upon common pitfalls and makes suggestions of how we can address them. We don't "do the program" merely by sitting and reading, it is a way to change our lives. A typical goal might be to work through a step a month. The timescale isn't that important and you can set your own goals based upon how quickly you want a good life. Move through these steps in sequence, read and fully understand the implications of what they propose. Take time to discuss them. The more we put in to this phase, the more we get out of it.

Living It- From today forwards you can start to live a new life free from drink and on the road to recovery. Dip into this section to see if the fears and problems you encounter are similar to those others have experienced.

Getting Started

What is Alcoholism?

A classic first issue is the word *alcoholic*. The word carries such a stigma that we could accept anything but – that word. Although it conjures images of park-benches, and old coats tied with rope - this is not the truth. It describes a person with a sickness that nobody asks to have (it is not self-inflicted). It afflicts people from all lifestyles. Those who treat it go on to lead perfectly normal lives.

Alcoholism is a killer illness. Worldwide, thousands die of it each year. It does not go away because we stop drinking; it waits and progressively gets stronger. During the period when we refuse to accept that we have it, we try a vast number of ways to remove the symptomatic problems. We change the style of our drinks, the time that we drink, the people we drink with and the places that we drink. We move house, change our partners and our jobs. We try religion, witchcraft, debauchery and piety. No matter what we change, the problems can decrease for a time, but they always come back.

Symptoms

Friends, family and doctors can tell us, but self-diagnosis is the only way that a person accepts that they have a problem and becomes willing to recover. Whilst there are a large number of symptoms exhibited by people who suffer from this illness, the following are extremely common ones. (This section has no medical basis).

Unpredictable mood changes, we swing from being happy, amusing and agreeable through to aggressive and depressed. The aggression can manifest physically, although it is more usually verbal and mental in nature.

Isolation, we have intense feelings of loneliness and feel cut off from the world. Even in a crowded place, we can feel alone.

Self-absorbed, we will frequently become "turned in" upon ourselves. We feel that we have problems that nobody else understands or can help with. At times, we will place excessive demands on those around for understanding or compliance.

Secrecy, we hide the quantity of alcohol we are drinking. If asked how much, we reduce the amount to what we feel is acceptable. We end up hiding empty bottles. We have feelings of guilt and shame, but we cover these from normal view by shows of bravado or aggression.

Consumption of alcohol, the quantity we consume varies from person to person, therefore as a means of diagnosis this is a poor indicator. A better indicator is the vehemence and indignation we display defending and justifying why drink is necessary. "Binge drinking", or life issues such as pregnancy or close medical supervision can mean that we go for many months without a drink. These interludes confuse and blur the issue for family and friends. People who love us cannot understand why, when we are dry, we are still exhibiting all of the other behavioural symptoms.

Prognosis

Without treatment, the sufferer will die of alcohol abuse, although the stated cause of death is often something else. Many verdicts of accidental death mask alcoholism. Walking in front of a car, or falling down stairs whilst drunk are common deaths for alcoholics.

Side Effects

The illness is contagious and spreads a secondary form to close family and friends. Even though they might not have joined us in our destructive drinking, they will exhibit confusion, anger, guilt and tiredness. The people closest to the sufferer carry a great burden of guilt and frequently require long periods of counselling and support for them to recognise and recover from the condition.

Treatment

There appears to be no cure for the illness of alcoholism. Once affected, the best we can hope for is to arrest it. This is what the twelve-step program does. The good news is that it works. A person who adopts and uses the program removes all of the visible signs of the illness and appears cured. The only person who needs to know that we are not cured is US.

In fact, it gets better than that. It is not just a return to life as we knew it, but a way to find a much more fulfilling one. All that we have to be aware of is that the monkey is always going to be there. The little rascal will whisper and manoeuvre in subtle ways to get us to take a drink. If we weaken and drink, we feed the monkey and give it the strength to take control again.

The Big Book and the Program.

The central book of AA is the "Big Book," it was from this book that the fellowship of AA took its name (the actual title being Alcoholics Anonymous). This book has helped many thousands of people rebuild their lives.

The founders set out to document exactly what they did to recover. This means that this book is like a workshop manual not a spiritual text. There are no hidden depths and meanings known only to the initiated. A workshop manual explains clearly how to do a job. For example, to remove the cylinder head from an engine it might read:

First, remove the air-filter by removing bolt "A" and bolt "B" and lifting the air-filter clear. Then remove the rocker cover by removing the four retaining bolts…

To some, the section above would be clear instruction on how to perform the task, but to others it is a meaningless string of words. If somebody explained it to us, we could do the job. The Big Book and the program are exactly this. They are clear instructions on how to return to an enjoyable and happy life. It is just that we sometimes need help to understand them.

What does hitting a rock bottom mean?

Is this the only form of illness where the patient has to get as sick as they can before they are willing to recover? This strange phenomenon is actually a symptom of addiction. Most people would rather get rid of a problem when they first notice it. If we have a stone in our shoe, would we walk on and hope it would get better by itself, or hope that nobody would notice us limping? Of course we wouldn't, we would fix it as soon as possible. However, for a much more serious problem, such as our life falling apart, it seems we live in hope that things will get better without us having to do anything drastic, certainly not stop drinking.

Every so often, we experience so much pain that we briefly gain an insight into what our life is actually like. This point is a "rock bottom". We often feel we have reached rock bottom when something dramatic happens and shatters our illusions. It is the point where for a moment we question if things are really going to be all right. Usually, it is losing something, a partner finally walking out and leaving us or losing our job.

There appear to be two styles of rock bottom; the first is a plummet, like a skydiver without a parachute. It is possible to descend from a point of feeling life is good, to not being able to face it in an incredibly short period, a matter of two to three months. The pain of such a descent is intense and we swear to ourselves that we will do anything to make sure that we will never feel this way again.

The other style of rock bottom appears to be more like a "trawler net" where the victim settles onto the rock bottom and then drags along in a state of pain and discomfort for a long time. Each rock and obstacle tears a small part of us away, whilst each new wound is painful, it remains justifiable and insufficient for us to stop and see how battered we have become. There are probably many reasons why people end up taking this route, certainly getting love and support beyond the point of deserving must be one of them. Yet another irony is that most illness responds when the patient receives attention and care, but apparently, the insanity of alcoholism doesn't.

The result of either path is a short window of opportunity where we reach a point of being desperate, the pain is too great and we are willing to do something about it. Too early, and we can still justify our behaviour and will not listen. Too late, and we are dead and cannot listen. It is always surprising how small this window is, but when it occurs, we might just listen.

Let's try to get the initial arguments out of the way...

People scouring this book searching for proof that they don't need to stop, will be able to find it. Paradoxically, only somebody with a drink problem looks for such proof. If the monkey can get us to accept that everybody else has it wrong then we remain under its control.

Nobody except ourselves can diagnose that we are alcoholic. This is something we have to do for ourselves. A good definition to help with this is:

If alcohol is causing a problem in any area of your life and you continue to drink you are probably an alcoholic.

Examples of these problems would be arguments with a partner, work problems, getting into debt. If it "costs" more than money, it is a problem that we would be better off getting rid of.

People raise a number of initial objections when they look at the program. The monkeys on our shoulders use exactly the same arguments and the symptoms are the same. This means that we have two internal voices raising queries and fears, our own and the illness. Our own fears are the natural concerns of somebody considering moving outside their comfort zone, but the suggestions placed by the illness are trying to stop us getting better.

Typical arguments

The main weapons that the illness uses to keep control of our lives fall into three main categories, Intellectual snobbery, Pride and Fear. It actually doesn't matter if the argument is real or imagined, the decision to get better means that we have to face these arguments and press ahead with recovery anyway.

We are scared that we will have too much to face, the illness has provided us with a buffer from reality and we have built up a bow wave of problems. Relationships lie in tatters. We know that we have creditors, both financial and emotional. The thought of facing these problems can seem frightening and too much to handle. We have all been through this. It takes time to put all of our affairs in order, but the mess is rarely as great as we anticipate. What the program offers is a way to put these issues into perspective and to resolve them as part of our recovery. We learn to stay away from drinking one day at a time and also to grow, recover, and repair our lives one day at a time.

We are scared that our family and friends will ridicule us, we believe we have a certain standing amongst our peer group. If we expose a weakness such as not being able to drink, or even worse, appear to be mixing with a strange religious cult, they are going to laugh at us. It is true that we do lose some of our friends, but we rarely lose anybody who matters. Anybody who thinks that it is shameful not to drink is probably not a good friend. Rather than base our future on what we imagine others will say, we could try the new way of life for size and then see how we feel.

We reject the ideas out of hand because they are old fashioned, It would be a lot more exciting if we could claim that this was an exciting new scientific discovery, or if it had been found written on papyrus scrolls, but we can't. There is a psychology that demands that we fix our problems using "new" techniques. This is why there is always a new diet, a new exercise regime or a new method of reaching our inner selves. We would feel silly if the answer to our problem had been there all along.

The principle of the AA program is an example of timeless resilience. Without a glitzy marketing campaign, it continues to grow and to save lives. Just like hands on a watch, it is a principle that works. We are dealing with a life threatening illness - <u>OUR</u> life. Put in these terms which should we trust, the latest "Fix your life in thirty days" scheme or a proven technique with over sixty years of success?

We reject the ideas out of hand because they are male oriented, Women frequently have difficulty with this and are defensive about their right to be recognised.   Nothing in the program infers that either gender is inferior. The program merely comes from an age when the obvious alcoholics were men. Naturally, women drank and died back in the thirties and it was far more socially unacceptable for them. We all suffer equally from the illness and it is important to remain focused on recovery. Can we improve anything by changing every gender related statement so that he/ she are used? Don't let gender snobbery get in the way.

We reject the ideas out of hand because they talk about God and Higher-Powers, few people adhere to a conventional religious faith and these can be challenging subjects for us to discuss. Recovery requires no religious affiliations whatsoever and it is certainly not a religious cult. We look at this subject in depth in step three. The program is spiritual in the purest and simplest sense, it is a way of being and fitting in. All that is required is to accept that we are not at the centre of the universe. Rather than abandon trying the program based upon a suspicion, it is better to continue, but remain cautious.

We sneer and reject it because it is a silly American idea, The objection could be as noble as "why is it the AA program? They can't even spell programme!" By tricking us into adopting a lofty intellectual principle, we slam the door on any chance of listening. If the illness can generate a pitying sneer from us, it has won. We reject the chance of recovery in the hope that we will impress somebody with our integrity.

We sneer and reject it because – (no reason, but we always sneer and reject) we often strongly belief that our own opinion is "right". Because the people at the meetings don't seem to adhere to our opinion, we judge them as wrong. These objections could be, "They don't have decaffeinated coffee", "they smoke", "they swear". By becoming critical of the defects, we become blind to the benefits.

They won't understand, I am a special case, We use initial knee jerk statements such as "I can't be an alcoholic, I don't drink as much as…" or "I have to drink as part of my job, I need to entertain customers". The illness wins if it can get us to justify the way we are acting.

And the point is?

If we have ever had to defend how much we drink, there could be a problem. People don't make these suggestions out of spite. If somebody close to us has challenged our behaviour, it was almost certainly because they don't want to see us destroy ourselves. We probably refuted it, creating fatuous reasons why they want us to stop. We think they are jealous or want to control us. We refuse to accept the need to change and wrap ourselves in righteous indignation at such a suggestion. We quickly move the focus from looking at our drinking into a discussion of their shortcomings. We can even pursue it further and turn such discussions around into trying to solve their problem and get them to see how flawed their thinking has been.

Even when we suspect that there is a problem, if the illness can convince us that we are the only ones to feel this way then it wins. One of the tricks the monkey plays is to isolate us. By keeping us isolated, we cannot find a way out. We never become aware that there are people who actually do care about us and can help us to get well. By making us feel alone we can justify our self-destruction. We long to cease to exist and dream of a solitary death, hoping to go to sleep, never to awaken.

What's the point, I saw that rock star xxx is back on the booze; publicity and the public downfall of high profile advocates allow the illness the freedom to mock and ridicule these failures. The monkey draws our attention to them in the press or on television. We justify that if they cannot manage to stop drinking after spending vast amounts of money on private clinics why should we even start the attempt. These public failures are extremely destructive and we discuss this later in the section on opinions. Once we know more about the program we are equipped to see how these celebrities have been tricked into relapse by the illness and how there really is a way to a new life that costs us nothing except a little of our pride. Remember that for every high profile failure there will also be a number of unmentioned successes. Many public and famous figures recover and keep the fact outside of the media spotlight.

Whilst we claim to be willing to look at things with an open mind, we usually look at the program with a closed one. We approach the investigation from a position of strong opinion and prejudice. By starting from a point of contempt, it is difficult to move on to a point of acceptance regardless of the facts placed before us. This is because we have the illness chattering in our ears, working to make us reject any concept of recovery.

Pride and fear interlink making it frightening to contemplate labelling ourselves as alcoholic. We are worried about what people will say and how they will react to us. Is this pride or fear?

We need to become confident that it is all right to investigate further because we can turn back at any time. There is no secret enforcer going to appear on the doorstep and demand that we attend meetings and get back on the program. The only commitment is the one that we make to ourselves. This is a commitment not to drink and to try to put the program into our life – just for today.

Why should I bother?

This is the thought of many as they approach the idea of adopting the program. To the rational mind, the promise of staying alive would seem sufficient. To those in need of the program this prospect can frequently seem abhorrent. We think that remaining alive means facing the demons that threaten us. We feel too frightened to consider facing life without drink.

If we approach this with unrealistic expectations or goals, we are setting ourselves up to fail. It is common to hold onto ideas like "I will do the program if it stops my Wife/ Husband from leaving me" or "I will do it if I can keep my job". The only thing guaranteed by working the program and adopting a new way of life is stopping drinking. It does not carry the promise of eternal youth or boundless riches. By staying alive, not drinking and adopting this way of living, many experience much more, but it is no defence against life. It cannot mend a broken leg or cure cancer. Life deals the cards and we have to work with them, but at least we know what game we are playing and can see the correct number of spots on them.

Most of us actually benefit by far more than simply staying sober for one day at a time. In the Big Book there is a short section known as the promises.

> *We are going to know a new freedom and a new happiness. We will not regret the past nor wish to shut the door on it. We will comprehend the word serenity and we will know peace. No matter how far down the scale we have gone, we will see how our experience can benefit others. That feeling of uselessness and self-pity will disappear. We will lose interest in selfish things and gain interest in our fellows. Self-seeking will slip away. Our whole attitude and outlook upon life will change. Fear of people and economic insecurity will leave us. We will intuitively know how to handle situations which used to baffle us.*

(Big Book Alcoholics Anonymous)

These promises don't come true as soon as we commit to doing the program. We earn them by progressing through it and they should begin to show up when we reach step ten.

What can we do?

If it were as simple as telling somebody to stop drinking, we would not need an organisation like Alcoholics Anonymous. Later in this book, we go into more detail about the meetings and support that contribute to our recovery. To recover we need to follow what AA suggests. Stop drinking, go to and take part in meetings, get a sponsor and work through the program.

Stopping drinking is extremely important – the program cannot work if we don't. We don't make a promise to stop forever we do it one day at a time. If one day seems too long, then stop for one hour. By going to meetings, we gain support and understanding. A sponsor is simply somebody to help us work through the program.

So without further introduction let's look at the beast. A warning before we do, it contains words that offend or affront. We will see potentially frightening words like God, Humility, and Change. Don't be afraid of them, they will all be explained as we proceed.

The 12 Step Program of Alcoholics Anonymous

(Big Book of Alcoholics Anonymous)

1. We admitted we were powerless over alcohol — that our lives had become unmanageable.

2. Came to believe that a Power greater than ourselves could restore us to sanity.

3. Made a decision to turn our will and our lives over to the care of God as we understood Him.

4. Made a searching and fearless moral inventory of ourselves.

5. Admitted to God, to ourselves and to another human being the exact nature of our wrongs.

6. Were entirely ready to have God remove all these defects of character.

7. Humbly asked Him to remove our shortcomings.

8. Made a list of all persons we had harmed and became willing to make amends to them all.

9. Made direct amends to such people wherever possible, except when to do so would injure them or others.

10. Continued to take personal inventory and when we were wrong promptly admitted it.

11. Sought through prayer and meditation to improve our conscious contact with God, as we understood Him, praying only for knowledge of His will for us and the power to carry that out.

12. Having had a spiritual awakening as the result of these steps, we tried to carry this message to alcoholics, and to practice these principles in all our affairs.

For some this is goodbye...

For many of us this is as far as we get. The illness is always present and is constantly twisting and manipulating our thoughts away from anything that will give us the strength to control it. Insidious thoughts seem to justify why following this path is not right for us.

If it is goodbye, I hope that you do not have the problem of alcoholism. Once afflicted, this illness does not get better. Regardless of whether we drink, it gets progressively worse. It is possible for people to put the drink down for long periods by will power or circumstance, but when they pick it up again they find themselves almost immediately at the point they left off and continue to descend farther extremely rapidly.

By accepting the possibility that the addiction works this way, we accept the first part of step one and have started on the path to recovery.

The Honeymoon period

Once we make the decision to try to sort our lives out using the program some of us experience a feeling of euphoria. We think life is going to be great and it can be, for a short period. Some talk about floating on a "pink fluffy cloud" for the first few weeks. Whilst there is nothing wrong with getting a feeling of well being, there are two pitfalls to watch for. It can trick us into believing that we have solved the problem and there is no need to progress any further. Secondly, when the high feeling evaporates we shouldn't allow the subsequent low feeling to convince us that the program is not working for us. If we proceed with the program, our life will improve and we recognise that the pink fluffy cloud was merely a superficial glimpse of the contentment that is to come.

Simple Checklist:

Am I willing to try to improve my life?

Am I willing to try to change?

If we can answer yes to both of these then let's journey a little further together.

Step One

We all remember the choice that occurs in horror films. There is a fork in the road and there are two paths. One of them looks dark but manageable, while the other one looks too forbidding to contemplate. The party wants to take the easier path, all, except for the native guide "There are bad things down that path, you need to follow me!" As we watch, we want to shout at them to listen and take the advice. We know that in their situation we would have listened to the guide.

It would of course be a boring film if the party reached safety by the quickest and easiest way. Good films involve tension, suspense and sometimes monsters.

When we reach the first step, we can see two paths and our native guide is willing to show us the easiest and quickest way to safety. What choice is there? People promise that if we work through these steps our life will improve – dramatically! The choice is a good film ending, or a real and enjoyable life. Think about it before choosing.

Many of us talk of having a film playing inside our heads. It plays slightly out of step with reality giving us time to say what we would have wanted to say, or it replays in a loop repeatedly highlighting our failings. We hope that we are the stars and that everything will work out in the end, but we feel detached and sometimes blind to what is actually happening. Everybody else can see that we are in debt, emotional pain and destroying the lives of those around us, but we hang on to the idea that things are going to improve. It is in the small gap created by hitting "rock bottom" that we can look at both parts of step one, admitting that they are true for us and accept that the path the guide is suggesting is the best choice.

Every journey starts with the first step and the program is no different. The best way to do the program is in order, a step at a time.

And so the journey begins...

We admitted we were powerless over alcohol — that our lives had become unmanageable.

Step one is our first glimmer of self-honesty. Up until this point, we thought that we were in control and made the decisions regarding our lives. If we suffer from alcoholism, we have been unaware of how much the illness subtly influenced our behaviour. What we thought was our own self-will proves to be the "will" of the illness.

There is a saying: when you find yourself in a hole – stop digging and this step is that simple, this is the point when we decide to put down the shovel and assess how deep the hole really is.

In this part of the book, we are going to work through the program. As we work through it, we are going to progress and consider each step. In fact, we are going to do more than break the program down into each step, frequently we are going to break the step down into smaller chunks and tackle the step in the smallest sections we can. For example:

We admitted we were powerless over alcohol

In this, we do not even look at the first step in its entirety, merely the first part of it. My experience was:

Towards the end of my drinking, every night followed the same pattern. I would leave work with good intentions, planning to go home, cook and maybe take a little exercise. Then as I started to cook, the thought of "just a little wine in the cooking," would occur. I would then realise that it would be a waste not to have just one glass whilst cooking, followed by the obvious need to have a glass with the meal and finally the requirement to round the night off with a shot of something stronger.

When I honestly looked at this, it became my first example of being powerless. Even on nights when I had promised myself that I would start a new healthy regime, I still took that first drink. Having taken the first drink the others seemed to follow, I do not even recall questioning what occurred, it just happened.

The first drink does the damage

Up until the point of taking the first drink, we can usually hold our behaviour together. Having taken the first drink then the second and subsequent drinks are inevitable. This is why we need to maintain a commitment to not taking that first drink and why the illness appears so determined to get us to take it. Once alcohol has entered our system, we become powerless over where the alcohol takes us.

We use the self-honesty mentioned earlier and look at how many ways we allow ourselves to take the first drink. It is only in retrospect or when we try to stop drinking that we become aware of how powerless we are. Up until this point, we possibly claim that it is just a habit when we stop for a drink at a particular time. We may create "acceptable" reasons to drink such as claiming that it is a family tradition to close the day with a gin and tonic. It is common to attribute medicinal qualities to alcoholic drinks such as rum and blackcurrant for a sore throat, whisky or brandy for a bad chest.

Because other people don't understand the feeling of a compulsion, they can't see anything wrong in encouraging us to "have a small one." The word addiction is another of those frightening words that triggers a response of denial. Nobody wants a label like addict and even those who have suffered because of our behaviour try to deny the truth of our illness.

A loving mother never encourages their heroin addict child into taking just a small fix to build up their strength, but many parents continue to make excuses for their alcoholic offspring. They will go to the shops to buy the drink that their child cannot get for themselves. Even members of the medical profession wax lyrically about the therapeutic benefits of a small glass of red wine and suggest that no possible harm could come from one.

The fact that we look for excuses to continue to drink should be a warning in itself. If we didn't have an addiction, stopping wouldn't be a problem. If we suspected that green beans were the cause of our life problems most of us could happily walk away from them without searching for an excuse to have just the one. Of course, we could argue that this is too simple an analogy and that there are wide ranging social reasons to drink not encountered in green bean consumption.

Honesty comes in as we knock over our excuses to drink.

I need a drink to face… This is a fallacy created by film and television – drink does not calm the nerves of a normal person. By drinking ourselves into oblivion, we don't increase our ability to cope, but we can lower our inhibitions so that the unacceptable becomes acceptable and by having lowered our standards, we create the illusion of coping.

When we start to face situations, we realise that we function better with a clear mind and come to see that we can't improve any life situation by approaching it with our faculties handicapped.

I need to drink with my clients. Even people who work in the hospitality industry discover that their clients are just as happy dealing with somebody who is sober. Certainly, clients are usually happier with this than dealing with somebody who sometimes goes over the top and becomes unpredictable.

My family would think I was being awkward if I stopped. We often feel that we know what other people will think or say and make decisions based upon this "mind reading trick". We might think that we are making a decision that will please them, but is this really what we are doing. Are we really only drinking to please somebody else?

When we make the decision to stop drinking then all of the reasons are simply excuses. When we are honest, we can see that we don't really drive better with a few drinks, we don't become more entertaining and we don't think more clearly.

...That our lives had become unmanageable.

Once the monkey drinks, it takes control and we become the audience of a slapstick comedy.

Just before I stopped drinking, I went to the mayor's dinner. It was a grand social occasion and I dressed to kill. During the evening I drank and laughed, I felt it was my responsibility to flirt with all of the men and leave the other women envious of my charm. It was after midnight when I spotted her. A middle-aged woman in an over-tight dress, her hair was partly free and her lipstick smudged. I remember thinking that somebody should tell her to go home. I then realised that I wasn't looking across the room, but staring into a huge mirror...

Another friend told how the hospital had brought him back to life from alcohol poisoning three times. He didn't believe he had a serious drink problem, because he only drank to be with his friends. The need to be sociable led him back into drinking situations time after time. He laughed and said he had no problem stopping drinking, but staying stopped eluded him. He loved his wife and children claiming that they were the most important people in his life. He was horrified at the suggestion that he would abandon them to be with his mates in the pub. He thought the idea that drink would take priority over them was laughable. The fourth resuscitation failed, he remained dead on the table after popping in for a quick drink and a chat.

Although these examples of a life being unmanageable involve drinking, not all of the examples we encounter do. Such as, our partner and our lover find out that each other exist. This type of situation creates intolerable pressure and we crave the release from worry that we believe drink provides. We try to resolve the issue so that we are not to blame. If only that interfering busybody hadn't told our partner, then everything would have been all right. We don't question our right to have a partner and a lover, but being found out annoys us.

Our landlord suddenly stops listening to the excuses and finally demands that we pay what we owe them. We feel that they are being unreasonable, because we may have spent the money on food. We possibly sacrificed our income to pay for somebody else to do something. We feel righteous indignation at somebody suggesting that we are the type that will not pay the bill, we just need a little more time and understanding to get around to it.

As well as specific situations, we can simply experience intangible feelings. It is common to contemplate running away. We start to hope that we won't wake up in the morning, or consider self-harm. The self-harm we plan might only be sufficient to gain sympathy and avoid something or it can be as serious as thinking of crashing a car secretly hoping that we won't survive.

This chaos feels like walking in treacle. We feel that every way we turn we encounter obstacles and difficulties. People and situations seem to be blocking our progress. We want to enjoy life, but how can we when so many things keep going wrong. In our path is everything from rabbit snares to bear traps and we are tired of it all.

At first, it can be difficult to accept that these problems are alcohol related. However, Alcoholism as an illness goes much deeper than being unable to stop drinking. The problems and feelings described above come from the "ISM" of alcoholism, (I, Self, Me). When we examine the situations that we have blamed on others, a common factor starts to emerge; our actions and desires created them.

Identification – The first weapon in our armoury

Identify means we recognise our behaviour in the behaviour of others. It is as simple as saying "Yes, I did that" or "Yes, I felt that."

When we identify we can see that other people were the same as we are and that they improved their lives by changing. We might also see that we could improve our life by simply accepting that they have a solution to the problem we have been trying to ignore.

The monkey fights back against identification in three ways, deception, justification and comparing. It is possible to read the experience of drinking each evening and say "yes I do that, isn't it a great way to spend an evening". Possibly, not the anticipated effect, but it could be the reaction.

Justification, with phrases like, "working the way I do I need to unwind when I get in." or "I need to forget the day and enjoy the evening." Justification arrives in our mind literally at the speed of thought. As soon as we question what we are doing, the answer is there - instantly.

Comparing, when we listen to somebody's story and the monkey places the thought, "I cannot have the same problem because I haven't done that." The incident itself is irrelevant. It might be going to prison, driving whist drunk, waking up in strange beds, but the reaction is "I can't be because…" nearly every one of us reacts this way until we run out of excuses.

Deception, with thoughts such as, "Alcoholics are homeless and drink from bottles wrapped in brown paper", and then we list through our material assets and wealth, we have a car, nice clothes and we only drink the best we can possibly afford.

When we compare we look for excuses not to change, when we identify we find proof that change is acceptable. We have to change, but won't until we break through the deception that the illness has used to disguise itself.

Breaking through to honesty

Discussion with somebody who has done the program is an excellent way to force ourselves to look at our motives and evaluate them honestly. If we take one of the examples given above, *our landlord is demanding their money*. Under these circumstances, we tend to be angry about how unreasonable they are. We might not have the money because we have had to cover some unexpected expense. If we took this problem to a friend in the pub, they would agree the landlord was being unreasonable and should be willing to wait.

If we take this to somebody who is actually listening impartially to us, the response could become a little more delving. How many times have we not paid in the past? When did we realise that we could not pay? Did we discuss this with them? We are not always in the wrong, but we tend to make decisions more in line with what we believe "should" happen, rather than considering other people. Unable to achieve our own agenda, we can become nervous and uncomfortable.

By having our behaviour challenged, we can see that the other person is reacting to a perceived wrong. Within AA we meet people who have done and thought the same as we have. When we give them the opportunity to listen to what we have been doing, they smile and recognise our veneer of justification for what it is. They know what we are thinking, sometimes before we do and can encourage us to take responsibility for the real motivation behind our actions.

<u>Writing things down</u> can also help. We can do this by making simple lists of situations that we have tried to control. Having made the list we can then look at them and work through noting what the result has been, for example:

I need love in my life.

My partner got fed up of the lies and kicked me out

I went to singles clubs, but each one was worse than the last

I had an affair at work and now the boss is angry

I think I am going to lose my job

By looking at the example honestly, we can see a progression through from deciding what is best for us and trying our hardest to achieve it. We originally see our "head down" determination to achieve goals as an asset. Whilst there is nothing wrong with ambition and goals, our attempt to impose our will upon other people often proves to be a liability.

There is no "right" way to break through to honesty. Both methods help us look at how we try to manage situations and how they seem to become more complicated. Sometimes talking with somebody else who is willing to challenge our motives works for us, sometimes, sitting and looking at the facts written down on a piece of paper is the only way we will accept that we have failings.

It is time to choose.

We started this chapter discussing the choice made in an old horror film. There are two paths. Both of the paths ahead may look forbidding, our current life is becoming darker and more frightening, but it is hard to imagine taking another route. The other path appears too strewn with obstacles for us to overcome. The guide assures us that we will be safe and that in reality it is the only path to where we need to go.

The experience of a rock bottom is fleeting and transient. For a single instant, we see that our way of life is not wonderful and that somebody else can show us a better way. If we let it pass, the monkey wins again, we soon laugh at the ridiculous idea that we would want to stop drinking.

What started the day as too horrific to contemplate facing again becomes another anecdote in our library of near misses. We appear to go around in a circle, but the circle is actually a descending spiral. On each spin we leave behind the good aspects of our life, as we descend, the unacceptable becomes acceptable. The person that claimed to have never woken up in a strange bed finds that it happens, then it becomes what they expect, eventually progressing to the point where they stop waking up in beds, but in bushes and public toilets.

By accepting the ideas in Step One, we are starting on the road to recovery. If we can answer yes to the questions, "am I powerless over alcohol?" and "is my life unmanageable?" then we are ready for a journey through the steps.

Step Two

I recall many years ago listening to a radio program whilst driving. The person on the radio was discussing at what point does an infidelity start? Did it start at the point of climbing into bed or at the first stolen kiss, maybe it was at the first confiding laugh, or perhaps with the first fleeting thought that accepted the possibility?

Looking at the problem of drink in a similar way, at what point does the first drink occur? Is it actually taking a drink? Did it start perhaps at the opening of the bottle, or when we took the careless stroll down the booze aisle at the supermarket, or perhaps in the first fleeting thought that accepted the possibility?

When it comes to manipulating our emotions the illness can play a "waiting game" and set us up for a fall a day, a week, or even months in advance of the event. If we review our behaviour, we can often trace the drink back to dangerous thinking a long time before the event occurs.

It is strange that we can be intelligent and controlled in much of our lives and yet keep finding ourselves in a mess. We sometimes have an impulsive urge to "press the destruct button". Our job might be going well, but we suddenly have to take our manager to task over something we consider a transgression of acceptable behaviour. We might have a loving partner, but abruptly decide that the relationship is wrong and they are not treating us the way they should. We inappropriately explode on these unsuspecting victims unleashing a deluge of ill feeling and venom that swamps the trust we have established.

There are times when we hurt people and we are surprised at their reaction. It seems that we don't fully grasp the normal "rules" of social interaction, or we believe that they don't always apply to us. We might claim to have been acting for their benefit and that it's not our fault that they misunderstood our intentions. Whilst alcohol is not directly involved, it is never far away. Because of "what we've just been through", we justify taking our emotions for a drink, losing sight of that fact that we triggered the situation that we are now bemoaning.

An alcoholic's life is full of reasons to drink. We think it's a virtue that we don't accept things tolerated by other people. We go to battle for our rights and the rights of others and we sometimes needlessly stir people up just to get a reaction. Although we have heard people mention serenity, we rarely listen to what they are really talking about.

If we are happy, we drink to make us happier, if we are sad, we drink to cover the sadness, if we are angry, we drink to calm us down and if we are frightened, we drink to bolster our confidence. Is there any other drug relied upon to answer so many situations? We might think we are special and different, but this fact alone indicates that we have an addiction. Any addict will tell you that they cannot function without their drug of choice.

When we accept that we suffer from alcoholism, we are accepting that the voice of the illness mingles with our own thoughts and where drink is involved draws us away from rational thinking. If we cannot trust our own thinking, we can accept the label "insane".

Came to believe that a Power greater than ourselves could restore us to sanity.

Within this step, we are facing two highly contentious issues. Masked behind the huge idea of a power greater than ourselves is the proposition that we are insane. Our "Intellect" screams that this is too much to consider and that we should not proceed any further. However, step two doesn't demand that we accept a "Higher Power" or even accept that we are insane. It is about considering ways to move out of our self-destructive rut and start to recover.

For some, the issue of accepting the existence of a power greater than us is a problem. Others arrive at AA confident that they have a strong faith, but the illness can even use this to trick us.

Because I had been involved with the church for years, I had looked at the program and quickly ticked off the steps I didn't need to do. I assumed that living a Christian life would cover most of the program. Step two looked easy, because I had no problem accepting a Loving God.

After a few months, I was floundering and I met up with my sponsor in a local café to talk. I thought I had done the program, but I felt lost. I assumed he would tell me it was normal to feel lost at this stage and we would laugh and have a coffee. Instead he produced the Big Book and asked me to read out the steps working backwards to ascertain where I was having a problem. As I reached step two I said, "Came to believe- been a Christian for years, done that."

He stopped me and asked me to read it again, I repeated myself, cursing the fact that he had obviously not been listening and he asked me to re-read it again.

Finally, to placate him, I read the entire step word for word and suddenly saw what he wanted me to acknowledge- that I was insane and unwilling to accept help. It seemed that "been a Christian for years" wasn't even close to addressing this step.

I was indignant. I had harboured fears for my sanity, but I had never shared them. I opened up and out cascaded a torrent of things that I had been trying to ignore. I rapidly acknowledged that regardless of my proclaimed acceptance, I didn't want to look at my behaviour and I didn't believe "outside" help could work for me.

It is now obvious that the step had ceased to exist, because I smugly assumed I knew what I was doing.

The program is a set of written instructions to get us from misery to miracle. Similar to the written instructions to get anywhere:

Leave home and turn left. At the end of the road turn left. Pass a road on the left and one on the right, turning left at the school. Follow the bends, but stay on the main road. At the end, turn right and turn right again. After the small warehouse turn right and go to the end. Pull into the car park on the right.

If we are following the instructions above and skip the occasional right or left turn, we won't end up turning into the correct car park. By attempting the program in isolation, we can easily trick ourselves into skipping over parts of it. It is safer if we accept guidance because this achieves three things. It keeps us safe, it teaches us how to speak honestly about our hidden feelings and helps us achieve a level of humility.

Came to believe...

These words seem to jump out and suggest a soapbox preacher demanding that we "see the light", but this is not the intention. It is as simple as, "came to believe that water would flow when we turn on the tap," or "came to believe that the kettle would boil when we switched it on."

We simply accept this to be true, but these are not common amenities for a person living in the heart of Africa. They would find it difficult to believe that these things would happen. They would need to try them repeatedly and be amazed that they worked before they finally came to believe.

Would it matter if they had used other words? Regardless of the exact wording, the step is challenging us to consider difficult concepts. The suggestion is that we need to look at a new idea and like the person in Africa who had never experienced having tap water before, we probably need to test it a few times before we start to accept that it works.

...that a power greater than ourselves...

What constitutes a power greater than we are? Gravity itself seems to be such a thing. Regardless of will power, we cannot hover even a short distance above the ground. Like King Canute, we cannot forbid the sea to flow around our feet, or command the sun not to rise tomorrow.

Do these examples seem silly and pitiful? More pitiful than:

> *Drinking, knowing that we will take our car onto the public highway threatening life and livelihood.*

> *Passing out whilst we are minding our young child.*

> *Continuing to take the first drink knowing that once we start we cannot stop.*

The drink itself proves to be a power greater than we are. We continually used will power or situations to control our drinking and failed. We are outnumbered, surrounded by a vast number of powers greater than ourselves.

All we need to accept is that there are powers greater than us that can influence our lives. We are often self-opinionated and stubborn in our belief that "our way is right". This step is about shattering this viewpoint and accepting that "something" greater than us can help us in ways that we don't yet understand.

...Could restore us to sanity

Imagine for a moment the classic cartoon scene of an asylum. A room full of men and women each with their hand thrust inside their jacket. They are all dressed as Napoleon. They look at each other, they can see the insanity around them, each knows that the others cannot be Napoleon and are therefore mad. They know, because they are the real Napoleon!

Few will get any identification with this, because it is almost impossible for us to see our own insanity until we have moved away from it. Are we insane we ask ourselves? Surely, all those other people are wrong.

Stopping drinking or understanding step two doesn't restore our sanity. The practice of the entire program and changing our lives does this. All that is required, is to open our minds to the fact that we can allow change to occur.

The answer to "must I change?" Is yes, we need to allow radical change to occur in our life. Returning to a state of sanity will be a fundamental transformation, what is unknown is what this will involve. Actively seeking change comes later in the program, now is not the time to worry about what is going to change as we return to sanity.

Summary Checkpoint

In summary, this step is a preparation for what is to come. We have lived our lives based upon our own ideas of right and wrong. In the past, we have had a great deal of difficulty with the idea that anything outside of us is going to be of any help. By admitting that we are not the central power in the universe, we are making a tentative start towards humility.   This step merely asks that we give up trying to fix ourselves and accept that something else can.

- Looking at the behaviour identified in step one - does it seem insane?

- Can we accept that something outside us could help us to recover?

If we can't answer yes to these, it doesn't mean that we cannot continue. We can come back and see if anything has changed after step three.

What form do these insanities take?

In the second step it is "suggested" that we have been (or are) insane. The word insanity is emotive and we usually think of it in terms of asylums and straight jackets. By having our attention drawn to the extreme we are allowing the illness to deceive us into comparing – "I haven't done that, so I can't be."

There are various reasons why we end up in asylums, some receive treatment to assist rehabilitation or for depression. Another option is a condition termed "Wet brain" (a layman's term for alcohol-induced dementia) where our short-term memory is destroyed and our brain becomes too damaged to function correctly. Whilst this could be where we end up, it doesn't start here and most die before reaching such extremes.

A definition of Insanity is, "something that is not sensible and is likely to have damaging results." Many an alcoholic will immediately argue with this definition asking who has the right to say what is sensible and go on to rant about "political correctness" trying to stop people having fun.

But surely, this is just me...

We sometimes experience disturbing aberrations like hallucinations or paranoia, but most of us justify our insanities as, "this is me" and sometimes go further – "...they have to accept me as I am". We rarely acknowledge that we could change from our behaviour if we chose to. It would be unusual if a single person exhibited all of the following examples of "odd behaviour", but most of us can identify with the motivation behind them.

Other people, in relationships, we expect "eccentricities" that we wouldn't tolerate to be accepted. We can demand attention, or paradoxically, yearn for people to realise that we need consideration, but remain unwilling to ask for it. Our self-centred approach to others shows up in convoluted ways. Our demands leave a trail of confusion and hurt amongst those who care for us.

Obsession, when we feel we "need" something and cannot readily obtain it, our bull terrier tenacity can drive us to extremes. We can ignore all normal moral behaviour to achieve our goal and feel proud of our ability to do so.

Isolation often becomes part of our lives. Sometimes, we

no longer trust ourselves in public, not knowing what we are going to do or say once we have had a drink. At other times, we feel threatened by something we cannot identify that is frightening and waiting for us. We can be isolated because we feel superior, or isolated because we feel inferior. The effect is the same – in our isolation it is easy for our thoughts to drift into dark and sinister places.

Suicide, our thinking drifts towards desire for suicide or death. We can switch instantly from being happy with life into hating every waking moment and seeking escape.

Seeing things, our insanities can eventually manifest themselves as seeing things that don't exist, not the fabled pink elephant, but possibly mice, insects and little people.

Being pursued, either by human or supernatural forces is quite common, we imagine that the car parked across the road is there to observe us, or notice that we keep seeing the woman with the green jacket. We believe that there are demons or ghosts trying to possess us.

I was nearly asleep when I noticed the rasping breathing close to the bed. I held my breath, hoping I was imagining it. The sound went on and I knew there was something in the room. I fearfully reached for the light switch and clicked it on. There wasn't anything there.

I armed myself with an iron bar and searched the house before finally accepting that I was alone. I clicked off the light and the breathing started again. I knew that it was evil and that it had come for me. I realised that possession explained many of the strange feelings I had been having over the last few months. I lay in the darkness cradling an iron bar, helpless and frightened, waiting for the final assault.

A more clinical view...

There is a psychological theory that proposes life is made up of small cycles (Gestalt Theory).

- The person is at rest

- The disturbing factor, which may be (a) internal or (b) external

- Creation of image or reality

- The answer to the situation, aiming at

- A decrease of tension, resulting in

- Return of balance

The common example used to explain the cycle is:

A person is sitting comfortably, they realise that they are hungry and this hunger moves to become the focus of their attention. They decide that making a sandwich is a good idea. Making and eating the sandwich addresses their disturbing factor and they can return to a state of balance until the next cycle occurs.

The theory proposes that an interrupted cycle leaves behind "unfinished business" and that we have a need to return to finish it. In the example, if the telephone rings whilst we are making the sandwich we handle the interruption by creating a new cycle and then once that is complete we return and finish making the sandwich.

The failure to return to finish a cycle causes feelings of stress and dis-ease.

The principle of this cycle is irrefutable, it is a well-respected foundation of psychology, but when we attempt to apply it to the life of an alcoholic, it becomes strangely disjointed. An alcoholic is rarely to be found "at rest", because we tend to be always doing something. Even when we appear to be sitting peacefully, constant internal turmoil occupies our thinking.

When we move on to creating the idea of what will satisfy our "disturbance", it can obviously be a drink, but it can also be something unattainable. Possibly a wonderful night out which ends with us meeting the person of our dreams, who will then sweep us away into a world of riches and pleasure. There is actually nothing more guaranteed to fail than aiming for the unattainable and so we guarantee ourselves a frustrated cycle that we are unable to complete.

This style of thinking seems designed to create a whole series of unfinished cycles and consequently we continually increase our stress and dis-ease.

What can I do?

The answer is DO NOTHING.

At an early stage in recovery, actively looking to make changes can be dangerous. If we do, we tend to focus on one specific factor and believe that if we correct it, life will become normal again, we are usually wrong. We look back and think that at some point in the past we could have made the decision not to become alcoholic. If only we hadn't suffered the trauma of a specific event then we would have been fine. This is one of the common misapprehensions about drinking. That there is a single cause which, once eliminated, will allow everything to return to normal. We find it difficult to accept the true single cause of our problems – Alcoholism.

This means that the search amongst the other life events is a distracting waste of time. If we suffer from alcoholism, we are probably incapable of making a truly honest appraisal of how our life has progressed. If we could be honest, we would probably see that there was no clear point where life changed over, there was no single traumatic event to blame, we had drifted gradually through being "mildly eccentric" into totally unstable, drink had been a constant part of things along the way, but actually quite a silent and stealthy companion.

Alcoholism is a threefold illness:

<u>Physical</u> – When we take a drink, it triggers a physical craving for more. The first drink does the damage. If we don't take the first, we cannot take the second etc.

<u>Mental</u> – We are certain that drink is the only thing helping us get through our problems, the mess gets progressively worse, but we won't give it up.

<u>Spiritual</u> –When we understand the term spiritual as used within the program then we understand how the alcohol renders us "spiritually bankrupt". We became withdrawn from life, obsessed with our own struggles and sorrows. If we gave time to others, we did so for reasons of self-gratification.

But if I just change...

It is normal to feel lost. We are challenging our basic principles of life. Even though people tell us not to make dramatic and instant changes, the monkey tells us that we have to do something immediately. If we can't get the advice we want to hear from AA we often turn to old and trusted friends. Although very few people actually know anything about alcoholism it rarely prevents them from having an opinion about what we need to do to tackle our problem.

For most people their understanding of alcoholism comes from films and television. Some of these fictional representations can be quite realistic, but they become distorted if reality doesn't match the time slot or the story line the writers wish to achieve. Nobody believes that watching hospital dramas enables them to perform operations. The same is true of trying to treat alcoholism based upon knowledge gained this way. Even so it is surprising that we do listen to the advice they offer – "accepting that you have a problem is the first step to recovery", "Self knowledge is the key to it…", "what you need is a holiday", "what you need is…"

If we were dealing with a minor ailment then it might be acceptable to try a few "home spun" remedies, but we are tackling a life threatening problem. Although people mean well and want to provide an easy answer, it is actually more productive to accept that we have a difficult problem and that we have to work hard to solve it.

The fact that we have the "symptoms" of a killer illness and yet we hope to cure it through ill-informed platitudes surely proves our insanity. There isn't a quick fix and it much more responsible to accept that we are going to have to learn how to handle alcoholism– one day at a time.

Surely, I will get better now I have stopped drinking.

If we return to our examples from the first step, we can see that we were powerless over alcohol and that life had become unmanageable. If we evaluate our behaviour the way an outsider would, we can see that they are likely to judge our behaviour as insane.

Once we have worked through the program and gained experience in living our life in a new way the damaging behaviour will diminish and seem to vanish for most of the time. We never entirely remove it and often the first indication that the monkey is planning a new assault on our sobriety is realising that our old thinking is back.

Step Three

We can think of the program as a racecourse with a set of fences to jump. Many see steps Four and Five as the Bechers (Beaches) Brook of the program. This is a famous jump on the Grand National course at Aintree. The surprise of Bechers Brook is that the ground drops away on the far side of the jump, so having made what appears to be an impossible leap it then becomes a frightening plummet to earth on the far side.

On a racecourse, the hurdles range from easy through to difficult. We have possibly anticipated that the fourth step will be one of the difficult ones. With our eyes raised, we rush forwards, failing to recognise the full implications of the third step. Step three is just as big a hurdle, the first two steps ask us to look honestly at our lives and recognise that we have been suffering from the illness of alcoholism. If we do this after hitting our rock bottom, we are usually willing to accept the truth. In step three, we start to take our first action towards correcting our behaviour.

Made a decision to turn our will and our lives over to the care of God as we understood Him.

It seems an impossible demand, asking us to surrender control of our life, especially if we don't accept the concept of a Higher Power working for us. The good news is that the prospect of this has appalled thousands of us, but we have managed to achieve it. If we break this step down in reverse order, we can accept each phrase before actually looking at it in entirety.

...God as we understood him

Many people have a working faith, but they have never

expected that their God would take an active interest in their daily lives. They feel challenged by the idea that a Higher Power could or would intervene for them. Such people usually find it easy to look at the evidence in their lives and to move towards accepting that their Higher Power is working for them.

People who once had a faith, but feel deserted by God are possibly in the hardest category. They believe they have proved that God doesn't exist and usually feel that it is impossible to give God "another chance", but by adopting one of the following suggestions, they can move forwards.

A common statement is some variation on "If you had seen (experienced / felt) what I have, you would know there isn't a God." These are of course wonderful sound bites, but our experiences are rarely unique. In fact, others maintained or even found a faith through similar experience and adversity.

Our problem might be as simple as feeling worthless. We might feel that no higher power could consider helping us because we are so pitiful. We can feel that our life up to this point has been so contemptible that no Higher Power worth the name would associate with us, or we over-dramatically declare God abandoned us.

Possible alternatives to God

A person who is comfortable with their concept of a God or "Higher Power" probably doesn't understand why we would ever consider needing to have a section like this. However, many feel that the word God is too offensive to consider, but they can usually accept one of the following alternative suggestions.

The population of a large portion of the world are

comfortable with the concept of ancestors being available to support in times of need. It is possible to use the idea of a loved one who has died to provide care and guidance. The thought of a parent, grandparent or a close friend can be both comforting and motivating. A slight shift in thinking moves them from a loving memory into a position where they can oversee and help.

It would take quite a closed mind to deny the existence of nature. The earth and its environment obviously work in some kind of harmony. We can see this from the placement of the earth in relation to the sun, the tilt of the axis that provides the seasons, the interlinked relationships between plants, insects and animals. There is a pattern and a "force" that wants life to flow in a correct manner. As much as possible, nature attempts to heal the damage done to it. There are many examples proving that nature does heal; the eyesore that was once a man made coal tip sprouts grass and becomes merged back into the surrounding landscape.

A fundamental of oriental medicine is that there is a flow throughout the body and that removing blockages and correctly balancing this flow allows a body to heal itself. The blockage preventing our recovery is our own opinion and we can change this. Once we have, this "flow" will try to correct imbalances within us. Can we let that happen?

If these suggestions and concepts of outside influence are not helpful, the undeniable solution is the power of the meeting. If we attend AA meetings with the intention of getting well, we will do. These people will guide and help us. They can provide support when we thought we could not go any further. If we grasp the first step of the program and attend meetings with an open mind, "something" removes the compulsion to drink.

Is it possible to deny that this is a power greater than we are? On our own, we could not stop, but with this help, we can. Possibly our oldest substitution trick is to use the (G)roup (O)f (D)runks in place of the word GOD.

...to turn our will and our lives over to the care of...

A misleading, but commonly used illustration of handing over is "letting go of the wheel", but surely it would be insane for somebody driving a car to do so. Possibly a better way of viewing this is to see ourselves as an interfering passenger reaching across and trying to wrestle control from the driver. Why would we do this?

Although we may deny it, many of us exhibit a nature that might be termed "Control Freak". We often become distressed unless we are able to control the situations and people around us. Sometimes we use subtle control by creating the environment that guides others towards our will. Sometimes it is brutal and we force and abuse those we want to control. Obviously, we don't do this to be cruel and we justify it by telling ourselves that we are acting in their best interests.

Our dilemma is threefold and is a difficult knot to untie:

- We are uncomfortable when we don't feel in control.

- We don't trust other people to get things right.

- We are told that we are not in a position to control our life.

By looking for examples in our past, we can see that handing over actually works. Here are two examples of being willing to hand over, one to a "God" and one to the Meeting.

The "God" example:

I came to the realisation that I could no longer live the life I had. My wife and children were gone, my job was at risk and I knew my sanity was in question. I lay in bed and cried. I looked up and said, "If there is a God then this is the time I need you, I cannot take any more."

Through an amazing sequence of events, I was at an AA meeting the next night, taking my first tentative steps towards a new life. To the best of my knowledge, this was the first time I had truly surrendered and asked for help. I had certainly never considered that AA might be an answer.

The Meeting example:

When I first started in recovery, my wife allowed me to see my children on Sundays. Each time I handed them back, I became distraught and wanted the oblivion of drink. One Saturday night I shared about this anxiety at a meeting. After the meeting, somebody approached me and suggested that until I became strong enough to cope I should stop seeing my children completely. My emotions screamed objections, the idea horrified me.

"Willing to go to any lengths" came into my mind and I accepted their guidance. For three months I did not see my children, we told them I was working away. I attended meetings and started to build a little sobriety. I genuinely feel that without this period of respite I would not have survived.

Other people's examples are rarely sufficient to convince us and we need to look honestly for our own. It would be unusual for somebody reading this to have lived a life without trauma. We can try to remember our lowest moments, the times when we thought there was no way out of our predicament. If we despaired and finally surrendered all hope, what happened? It is possible to see how "by coincidence" a chain of events resolved the problem. There might only be one or two incidents, but this should be sufficient to kindle a glimmer of faith in something bigger than we are.

Made a decision...

What is a decision? We make hundreds of decisions every day, we are not even aware of most of them. We feel that we are good at making some of them, but others leave us feeling uncertain.

In simple terms, we make decisions by allowing a number of factors to "vote" and we then act upon the result of the election. Examples of these factors would be, like and dislike, comfort and discomfort. These factors are the thoughts that occur constantly throughout the day, sometimes they scream at us, but at other times they might be subconscious and we are not even aware of them. The monkey also tries to influence the vote, certainly on anything to do with alcohol.

A simple example of the decision process occurs when we are leaving the house. We need to decide if we should take a coat with us. To do this we take all of the information we can and allow the vote to occur. Where are we going? What is the weather like and what is it likely to be in the near future? If it is cold and raining, our desire for comfort outweighs the dislike of the extra burden of a coat, guiding us into making a decision. Making a decision baffles us when we don't have sufficient information to allow the voting to produce a clear choice.

In the first steps, we gathered information about our

current situation:

- We are powerless over alcohol

- Our lives are unmanageable

- We are suffering from insanity

- There is help if we ask for it

Now we can add another piece:

- Our life based upon "self" has brought us to where we are.

In the past, we have used a positive view of our "self" orientated life perceiving it as "self"-reliance and "self"-sufficient, but probably ignored the negative implications such as "self"-centred and "self"-seeking. This additional information indicates that we cannot trust ourselves to make impartial decisions.

When we consider all of the facts, we see that we are not equipped to make our own life decisions. This means that the only sensible decision is to stop interfering and hand this process over to the "God" that we trust.

Putting it all together

Made a decision to turn our will and our lives over to the care of God as we understood Him.

If we have understood and accepted each of the individual phrases in the step, it suddenly becomes much easier to accept.

How exactly do we hand our lives over?

Even if we are still convinced that there is "nothing out there", we don't lose anything by saying a prayer asking for help each day. We have made a great start if all we do is confirm to ourselves that we want to live our life without imposing our will during the day.

When we encounter a specific problem, there is no better way to demonstrate humility than with the simple statement, "I give up". We can then mentally "commit" the problem to our higher power. The next action is to share the problem with other members of AA as soon as possible without trying to lead them towards our preferred solution. We can then stop trying to resolve it for ourselves and get on with things that do concern us. If we find ourselves once again attempting to resolve the problem, we simply repeat the process of handing it over and sharing about it.

This is of course easy to suggest, but extremely difficult to achieve, the thoughts can creep in at any time and we sometimes need support in handing over our problems. Visualisation is one way that works. Imagine taking the problem and wrapping it up in a blanket. Visualise placing this bundle on the table at the meeting and humbly asking the meeting to take it away. Hold this picture for a time and "watch" as the bundle opens and the contents evaporate. This visualised activity moves into reality by sharing honestly about the efforts we are making to have our defect removed.

Keeping it in place

It seems unimaginable that we would discover a way to improve our life only to disregard it at some point in the future, but most of us find it difficult to keep these principles in place. Over time, we take back the control and guidance of our life and we literally seem to forget to hand things over to our higher power.

We will never be perfect and there is no reason to give ourselves a hard time for allowing this to happen. If we are practising the rest of the program within our life, we detect the drift before there is too much harm done.

A typical indication that we have taken back control is that we realise we are in conflict with those around us and nobody seems to be doing what they should. By recognising this thought, we can see that we are judging the actions of others and assuming that we know better than they do what should occur.

The more we try to control, the less satisfaction we experience in our lives. We become frustrated and we finally start to think about alternative ways to remove the difficult feelings. Thoughts like this prove that the illness is active and cunningly trying to draw us back towards drinking.

Summary

With step three, we decide that we will stop grasping for the steering wheel and allow a power outside of us do the driving. This allows us to look out of the window and enjoy the ride. If this all makes sense, we have successfully completed step three and started to construct a new and successful life.

Summary questions

This is a major checkpoint. Anybody who successfully reaches this point within the program has already progressed a long way into recovery. Remember that we don't have to make firm decisions regarding our Higher Power or God. We can switch our thinking to whatever idea works for us.

- Can I honestly identify an acceptable concept of a Higher Power?

- Am I willing to hand over control to this Higher Power?

Spiritual Paths

Like any good guidebook, we should consider the
suitability of the suggested paths. Only an irresponsible
guide would take infirm clients along trails appropriate
only for super fit athletes. Different people need different
routes and it is wrong to infer that there is only one correct
spiritual path.

The last step asked us to identify a God or Higher Power
that we could accept. In the next step, we are going to be
looking at "moral" defects. Both of these are intensely
personal challenges and don't need to conform to anybody
else's opinion. One person's moral behaviour is another
person's taboo. The final decision of what we are willing
to accept is ours alone, but we may take guidance from
people we trust.

At times, even accepting guidance can be dangerous. In
selecting a person to turn to, we risk giving the monkey
too much power. We allow it the opportunity to guide us
towards dangerous people. People can be dangerous
because through their guidance we end up pursuing a
dead end, they possibly say what we want them to, or not
understanding our illness, they enable us to remain
deluded. There are also people who prey on the
vulnerable, hoping to capitalise on weakness and we can
be too willing to listen unconditionally to their
suggestions.

The vicar's wife said that I would get the strength from God to
control my drinking, so I don't need to come to meetings
anymore.

It seems unlikely that a vicar's wife would have sinister
motives, but the monkey does. It constantly fights to drag
us away from recovery. It whispers, "Don't listen to those

people talking about the program, let's go and see if there are better routes to go down, they look easier and more interesting."

The "Big Book" warns about looking for easier softer ways that don't exist. It is also possible for us to invent harder and more difficult ways that don't exist either. We are starting to change and it tends to be around this point in our development that we become confused and lose sight of "Keep It Simple Stupid" (KISS).

If we look closely at the principles of the program, we can possibly identify Christian undertones. However, anybody with knowledge of any of the major religions of the world could identify influences from them as well. AA is not a religion and it doesn't matter one way or the other if we are or aren't part of one, it works for anybody who is willing to accept a "spiritual" way of life.

Not all spiritual paths are religious, but all religions are spiritual paths. If we look collectively at the major religions, Christianity, Islam, Hindu, Sikh, Buddhism and Judaism there are some specific guidelines that start to appear. The positive aspects of all of these paths suggest words like compassion, charity and respecting other people. The negative traits they all identify as dangerous are pride, envy, greed, lust and anger.

Rejecting these suggestions simply because we have an aversion towards religion seems pointless. In doing so, we are looking for the intellectual argument that will allow us to reject the program or seeking that elusive shortcut.

Some of us are tempted to return to our childhood religion because we think that it will help us with the praying and spiritual parts of the program. "Grab a fix, any fix" and move on as quickly as possible is a symptom of the illness.

Told that we should grow spiritually, we half listen and dive headlong into the past. We justify it by claiming that we are, "Going back to our roots". We visualise pictures of happy times and think we are receiving guidance back to the correct path. Having become engrossed in our "new found" spirituality we drift away from AA and present the monkey with an easy victory.

If we are part of a religion, or find one after stopping drinking, we remain safe if we keep it separate from the program and allow space for both of them in our life. If this is the first time we have been attracted to religion, before becoming committed to it, we should be consider the suggestion of not making any major decisions on our own for the first two years.

Understanding the word - Spiritual

Some of us react rather like a vampire to a cross at the suggestion of a spiritual way of life. We possibly indulged in the more sordid aspects of life, or we believe ourselves too intellectual to consider such superstitious rubbish. It is important to acquire an acceptance of the term "spiritual" that does not get in the way of progress through the rest of the steps.

A dictionary definition of spiritual is:

Related to the human spirit as opposed to material or physical (Oxford English).

This means that we cannot measure it by any of our senses: sight, smell, hearing, touch and taste. We can "feel", or strongly believe, but we can never actually prove the existence of the spiritual.

The basis can be as simple as becoming "needed, wanted

and loved". By using these simple guidelines, we can move gradually towards a spiritual way of life, possibly through the concept of "wholesome" living. Wholesome is certainly not a word that we would normally apply to ourselves in the latter stages of our drinking, but it describes four attributes for life that are worth considering.

Wholesome action is not harming others. Possibly, refraining from sexual misconduct and avoiding selfish behaviour.

Wholesome speech is not being offensive, gossiping or chattering meaninglessly.

Wholesome livelihood is earning our living in a way that does not harm others and looking for meaning and contribution into their lives through our work.

Wholesome effort is giving time to develop positive aspects of our lives and moving towards a more spiritual way of life.

All of the major faiths of the world propose similar concepts and we will change if we live by them. Hesitantly, we start to experience small pools of happiness. We realise that serenity is not boredom and reverse our understanding of life. Originally, gaps in the chaos were the low times, but as the gaps become contentment, our tolerance for chaos diminishes and we start to understand spiritual growth.

Moral Defects – What are they?

On the descent into the last painful stages of alcoholism, our boundaries of acceptable behaviour became blurred and as we recover, we need to re-learn appropriate behaviour. A good definition is:

Moral behaviour is not what we do, but what we refrain from doing.

Anger, Pride, Lust and Greed have appeared in the earliest spiritual writings as the cause of degenerate behaviour. We can usually identify anger or lust, but can mask defects such as greed with other intentions. There is nothing wrong with wanting a comfortable life, but we can easily slip over into greedy or gluttonous behaviour. Masking makes it hard to identify where our defect truly lies. If we can't recognise them and see how they have twisted our behaviour, we won't recover.

Listed below are common examples of how we remain chained to despair through our beliefs. It is our choice to hold on to the defects, or to work through the program of recovery to become free of them.

Do you want to keep – Fear?

Alcoholics talk of a racing brain and we seem to perceive frightening things that others don't. We are shocked when people leave their front doors unlocked, their cars with the keys in, or a baby left sitting in the back seat. To us these things are invitations to doom and disaster.

Where others carry on seemingly unaware of the potential for misery, the terror our imagination creates leaves us transfixed. A door left unguarded for a moment heralds the entrance of a marauding psychopathic gang from hell. Criminals will use our stolen car in a violent robbery and the police will link us to the crime. Bad things happen, we read of them every day, but alcoholics seem to be more aware of and act upon fears without stopping to find out if they are real or imagined.

We have fear designed into our being. In the wild, it is correct for a weaker animal to feel fear and flee at the sound of a strong carnivore heading towards them. In modern life, fear is still a valid response in some circumstances. If we have harmed somebody with power over our lives, such as stealing from our boss, then it is correct to feel fear.

We discover that our unhealthy fears become progressively more irrational. This doesn't happen suddenly, but creeps up on us like a strangling weed. We can't understand why we are scared, but we know that we are. We don't recognise it, but the monkey on our shoulder is incessantly chattering reasons to be frightened. It creates a continuous private showing of the worst horror movies we can imagine and we start to react to them. People frequently share that they slept with a knife under the bed, or could not answer the door without a baseball bat, or a shotgun concealed close by.

Do you want to keep – Projecting?

My sponsor told me to try an experiment. Take a deck of cards and shuffle them, hand them to somebody and ask them to turn cards for me to guess. I didn't do well, although I had always believed that I knew what other people were thinking – I didn't.

The same applies to the ability of projecting a future situation. We pretend that it is planning when we play the "they say - I say" game, but it isn't - it's projecting. We need to accept that we cannot predict the future and that we have to be able to handle life as it comes, trusting that we will be able to cope as it unfolds.

There is a difference between projecting and planning a future. Projecting, is when we operate our thoughts like a film projector and we project our thoughts and desires onto those around us. If people stand up in front of a film projector, they reflect a distorted section of the film. When we project, we see a reflection of our thoughts, not theirs.

Planning is, "I am going on holiday in five days and need to make sure I have the correct clothes to take with me", or, "I have a bill to pay and I need to save money to cover it". The difference is that planning sounds like something for people with boring lives. With the aid of projection, we can live on the edge and have fights with strangers, both verbal and physical without moving from our chair.

Do you want to keep - Living with resentment?

Living in the day is one of the throw away lines that people use in AA. To a logical person, it would seem quite difficult to live anywhere else, but for us it is actually the last place our mind spends much time. We are either looking at past victories, or more likely past failures. We dream of how everything will be better when "X" happens. "X" could be anything, like, getting a new job or the United Nations Security Council finally realising that it needs our help.

A strange fact is that although we could use the revisiting of past times for pleasure, we rarely do so. We could use the imagining of future times to visit a wonderful fairyland of happiness. We start our journey there, but quickly descend into hurt and hatred.

Life creates a set of oil paintings, fixed and unchangeable. When people look at their past they review these oil paintings, they can see good parts and flaws. However, the alcoholic wants to climb inside the frame and change what they can see. We try to paint over painful scenes and re-draw them to portray ourselves in a better light. Sometimes when we replay these incidents, we become locked rigid, every muscle in our body tense as we re-live an insult or embarrassing time from the playground or workplace. We recall our pain and inability to act appropriately, but then we go on to imagine how we would like to have reacted and made our tormentor suffer, we gloat at their pain.

There are many ways to phrase this concept, "once the page is written it cannot be re-written," "don't let people live rent free inside your head." Try as we might, we can't go back in time and undo anything.

Do you want to keep - Selfish Behaviour?

Our thoughts and motivations try to put us at the centre of everybody's universe. We cover it well, pointing out how we help others, but this is often a subconscious need to be indispensable. At other times, we are less complex and regardless of the impact, simply demand the attention we believe we deserve.

We know how much harm a drink will cause, but we still decide to take it. Even the suicide we imagine as a release for our family is actually the ultimate selfish act. Our own need overrides every other consideration. In our darkness do we honestly consider the impact our death would have, or do we secretly gloat at the guilt we would leave behind?

Do you want to keep – Allowing "if only…" to rob you of happiness?

We spend huge amounts of time in the fantasy world of "if only…" we have dreams of becoming rich and powerful. We think that the world will come to us. We waste large parts of our lives in an imaginary land where we have taken centre stage and have proved ourselves equal to the task. In every circumstance, we can see what is required and feel continually frustrated by the obvious failure of others to understand our plan, if only they would ask.

If only, can also lead us into looking for "quick fixes", such as, "if only I lost some weight, I would find a new partner", or, "if only I could pay off these debts, I would be able to spend more time on my sobriety."

We imagine that we know the solution to our problem and can justify bending the rules "just this once" to achieve our goal. The quick fix rarely works and we end up frantically applying sticking plaster upon sticking plaster to staunch the wound we have inflicted upon our life.

There is another side to this little phrase and this is the concept of creating Hell on Earth. It is easy to take a pleasant situation and by the slightest shift in thinking, remove the pleasure. For example, an excellent Sunday roast, ruined because there is no horseradish sauce. A day by the sea, spoiled because there was no ice cream. The simple utterance of "If only there had been…" reduces the pleasure.

The destructive powers of the phrase "if only," should never be under-estimated it creeps in to many aspects of our lives. By looking for the last iota of pleasure, we remove the pleasure that was actually there.

Do you want to keep - loneliness?

We drink ourselves into a state of isolation whether we are the over-confident extrovert seeking ever-brighter lights, or the uncertain introvert attempting to fit in. Unknown or real fears dominate us and we end up alone.

This is not the content aloneness and peace of meditation.

It is the hard to confess loneliness of a frightened child. We cover it with the bluster of phrases like "I am a lone wolf", "I am completely self-sufficient, I have no need of others". We feel abandoned by friends and family, as our life spiralled out of control they chose not to follow. We all take different routes along the descent, but the result is the same, isolation and loneliness.

We all drifted into the local throughout the day. By early evening, I would be sitting amongst a crowd of "friends". At some point, I would change. It was as if a bubble descended over me and cut me off from them. I could hear the conversation, but couldn't readily join in. My judgement of them was spiteful. Her laugh could shatter a glass and his skin made my stomach churn. I stayed, but felt apart. I sometimes joined in to show them how to tell a joke or have a good time, but when I reached home, I wept for companionship.

Do you want to keep – shame?

To feel shame is to feel seen in a painfully diminished sense. The self feels exposed both to itself and to anybody else present. It is this sudden unexpected feeling of exposure and accompanying self-consciousness that characterises the essential nature of the affect of shame. (Kaufman 1993).

The subject of shame is extremely complicated, it is a normal controlling emotion, but the interplay between fear and pride means that it is one of the monkeys' strongest weapons. Why do so many alcoholics hide the bottles that they empty? We proclaim that we are not doing anything wrong and aggressively defend our right to drink at any time, but feel that our behaviour remains acceptable on condition that nobody knows about the excesses. We can find ourselves in a vicious circle fuelled by shame. By drinking secretly, we drink more destructively. We sober up feeling shame regarding our actions. We vow that we will start to sort ourselves out and then we drink again to take away the feelings.

Many people are ashamed of incidents in their history. An alcoholic will almost certainly collect their fair share. Some of us spent a great deal of time functioning in a blackout (a condition where we appear to be coherent, but we have absolutely no recollection of what we do). Through lost inhibitions, we do things that we would not normally do. We also use the excuse of having a drink to justify outrageous behaviour. We can do whatever we feel like doing regardless of how unacceptable it is and claim that the drink made us do it.

The nature of these incidents varies for all of us, we possibly recall them boastfully, or we may suffer a stomach-churning wrench each time we recall them, sexual transgressions, physical, or mental abuse, bed-wetting, or the continual downward spiral of uncontrolled drinking. The common factor is that we wish they had never occurred and hope to take them with us to the grave.

Do you want to keep – secrecy?

As a practising alcoholic, there are so many secrets to keep hidden. Where have we been? Who were we with? What were we doing? There is the obvious secrecy that goes with alcoholism, hiding and covering up how much we drink. Our family becomes vigilant and comments if the bottles empty too quickly. In response, we become cunning. Whilst the bottle they can see doesn't seem to empty, the one in the garage / washing basket / garden shed, needs replacing far more frequently.

There are shameful incidents and the crippling need to

keep our fears secret. Many of us experience panic attacks, becoming scared in a supermarket or feel threatened in a crowded room. Having never put a label on the feeling, or discussed it, we believe that we are the only person to feel this way and cannot reveal it.

Finally

We are now working towards a full and successful life and we only achieve this by doing much more than stopping drinking. We are going to remove the thinking that allows the monkey to keep us under control. We are pushing the illness out of its comfort zone and it is snarling at our temerity.

The thoughts we may experience at this point will be things like:

- Now we have stopped drinking everything will get better. It is common to claim that we only wanted to stop drinking and don't want to change anything else in our life.

- We feel that because we are smarter than most people are, we don't need to go to the same extremes to get well.

- We claim that we are not as "sick" as they are and so we don't need to do as much to recover.

- We suspect that once we start to delve into and expose our defects, other people will not want to know us.

With these thoughts, the illness is using pride and fear to push us back into isolation and misery.

Step Four

We can imagine the steps of the program as a building process, with each of the steps contributing towards constructing a new way of life. In the first two steps, we decide our "house" is flawed and that it needs rebuilding. In the third step, rather than trust ourselves, we appoint an architect to oversee the construction. We need a solid foundation and in the fourth step, we are going to evaluate the structure and decide what to keep and what to get rid of.

Made a searching and fearless moral inventory of ourselves.

There are two main fears that hold us back when we consider doing this step. Fear that once we have completed it we have to reveal the contents to somebody else and the solemn warnings in the Big Book about failing to do this step thoroughly. We can be frightened that we won't remember all of the incidents we "should", so that through no fault of our own we won't correctly complete the step. There is a difference between actually forgetting and feigning memory loss. Providing we are determined to be honest as we approach this step, we will do it right. We can sort out forgotten incidents later, but skipping inconvenient ones can prove fatal.

Throughout this book, it has been emphasised that we do a step at a time in the order they are written. The same as building a house, the walls come before the roof. It is essential to ignore the remainder of the program until we complete step four – especially step five.

This is an "action" step. One, two and three are replacing old beliefs with new ideas. In the fourth step we do a specific task…

Made a searching and fearless...

It is important to recognise what the defects are and how they caused harm to others. It is easy to say, "I am too proud", but it is harder to describe specifically how our pride has led us into doing wrong. Pride and fear can be difficult to separate, is it pride or fear that stops us being able to play successfully with children because of what others might say? Which defect stops us speaking out when we see somebody victimised or injured by gossip? What forced us into spending more money than we could afford?

Many defects start as acceptable behaviour and in the Twelve Steps and Twelve Traditions it suggests that we suffer from "twisted instincts", where normal instincts have evolved into abnormal demands. There is nothing wrong with taking a well-earned rest, but this can become lazy behaviour. We try to justify it, but in our hearts, we know that we are shirking responsibility and putting extra burden upon others. We tend to be people who always want more - more food, more sex, more gratification, more... anything that gives pleasure.

The idea is to go through a process of detailing our hidden secrets and putting them down on paper. Times we harmed, cheated and deceived others. By getting the skeletons from the closet and re-visiting our feelings, we look honestly at why we acted the way we did.

...Moral inventory of ourselves.

Imagine for a moment that we are going to help somebody sort out a garden shed, its locked door has remained unopened for many years and nobody knows what is inside. It could be tempting to assume that it is all rubbish and throw the whole lot out, but then we won't see the hidden treasure that we are in danger of losing. We need to empty it completely, spreading the contents in the sunlight so that we can see what is there.

We would probably start to group things into piles as we lifted them out. We would put tools, tins of paint, and garden ornaments into separate piles for more detailed examination. By grouping the items together, it is easy to see that there are three garden rakes. Two of them are broken, but we can clean the third and return it to the shed.

The moral inventory we are embarking upon is a similar exercise. The shed is our life, full of our past behaviour and beliefs. Whilst the contents will emerge in a random order, we will find it easier to start to "pile" the contents into headings of a similar nature. In the last chapter, we suggested headings that we could use to group our defects. These are usually words like Anger, Pride, and Resentment.

How do we do it?

People often say that Step Four is where life started to get better. It is about preparing to build a new and solid life. Each defect we identify is a step out of the shadows towards the sunlight of contentment. Despite these assurances, we would not be human if embarking upon a deliberate examination of the worst parts of our character did not frighten us a little.

Although there are a few ways of doing the fourth step the best starting point is to try the method described in the Big Book using the three suggested columns.

Big Book Method

This method leads us to look at who or what we resent. We then dig down to the cause of the resentment and clearly state how this affected our feelings and life. From these roots, most of our defects seem to manifest.

I Resent	The reason I resent	This affects
Mr. Normal (My Boss)	He is not a bright as I am, but he is my boss. He will not listen to my advice I have to work hard to make up for his failings	Self Esteem (Pride) Personal security (Fear)
Mrs. In-law (My wife's mother)	She does not think I am good enough for her daughter. She does not believe a word that comes out of my mouth. I am scared that she will turn my wife against me	I feel insecure and threatened (Fear)
Mrs. Ex-Wife	She rejected me – she won't have me in the house. All of our friends have stayed with her	Self Esteem (Pride) Security (Fear)

An additional way of using this layout is to change the word "Resent" and use the words Angry and Frightened. Sometimes similar names and feelings occur, but when we do this, we open another rich seam of thought. The important part is to get the names of the people and the detail of why they make us feel the way we do. We need to be rigorously honest and have no fear about the fact that we will be discussing the contents with another person. Each incident from our past that causes our stomach to churn is usually associated with these simple headings: Resentment, Anger and Fear. Frequently the target or victim of the emotion does not deserve the venom directed at them and it often eases when we can accept our part in the situation.

Life Story Method

Some people write a life story, they work through the events of their lives and see their part in the situations they remember. This is a good way to build a framework and reinforce the fact that drinking is only a symptom a deeper illness.

Throughout our life, regardless of the advice of others, our selfish motivation drove us into foolish decisions. Incident after incident highlights how we attempted to control others into doing our will. As we chronicle our progress, it becomes obvious that many of the incidents occur well before the time we thought drink contaminated our life.

Two distractions commonly occur when we use the life story method. The first is that we can become embroiled in re-fighting past battles and reliving the arguments we believe we should have handled differently. Instead of writing, we spend hours transfixed by the tableau we create, indicating that we have allowed the illness to trick us into taking other peoples inventories, rather than concentrating on our own.

A second problem is that we start to imagine our life as a good novel or a gripping film. We cast ourselves as the angst-riddled hero of the tale trying to do the right thing, misunderstood, suffering and driven into desperation by a killer illness. We dwell on the mood lit camera shots highlighting our bewildered misery and meander away from honestly documenting what occurred into dramatic justification.

By avoiding these pitfalls, many successfully use the life story method to prepare their step four. Removing justification from our thinking is a great way to practice humility and teaches us how to live honestly amongst people.

Two Column Method

This is where we write two columns labelled assets and defects and put entries into each column.

For some strange reason we can decide that each column should contain a similar number of entries and frantically try to balance the columns. When we do this, we are confusing two issues, low self-esteem and a moral inventory. We are performing a moral inventory, our focus is upon the defects and it would be peculiar if we listed as many assets as we do defects.

We will address our self-esteem by completing the program and are possibly not yet equipped with sufficient moral judgement to be able to label all of the elements of our behaviour as an asset or a defect. As we progress and become more honest, behaviour we thought to be an asset can prove to be a defect. In the Asset column we might write, "I can always be relied upon to do any task I am asked to do". As we learn to look more objectively at our behaviour, we often change our mind. We realise that we should have written in the defect column, "I will do anything to please other people," or "I have to be the centre of any activities so that I am seen as indispensable."

If we become stuck trying to make these decisions, it is worth remembering that we don't have to complete step four in solitary confinement. It is perfectly acceptable to ask for help sifting through the assets and defects to assess them correctly. Our sponsor can listen to how we see our behaviour and point out where we are being lenient or harsh upon ourselves. Learning to rely appropriately on other people for guidance is an important lesson to learn and this is a good opportunity to practice.

Summary:

When we embark upon step four, it is essential to keep the fourth and fifth steps separate. Step four is preparing an honest moral inventory of our wrong doings and motivations. Once complete, in any form that we are content with, we have to get rid of all of the rubbish as soon as possible.

When we started our fourth step, the fifth was frightening, but as we reach the end we can get a burning urge to progress and do step five. If this is not the case, possibly we are still holding on to things, hoping to keep them secret. It cannot be emphasised too strongly to get these steps completed as thoroughly and quickly as possible, leaving hidden secrets to come back and trip us up later is probably one of the most common reasons for failing to achieve a worthwhile sobriety.

- Set a date to do step five and then ignore the fact that we will discuss what we write down with somebody else.

- Choose a method and allocate sufficient time to do it.

- Go to as many meetings as possible and talk to people that we trust.

- Do not hold anything back for fear that it will shock.

Step Five

In step four, we created an open wound by honestly probing our past behaviour. Step five will start the healing process. We are putting ourselves in danger if we procrastinate over continuing. Exactly like a physical wound, this one can lead to pain and death if it remains untreated.

Admitted to God, to ourselves and to another human being the exact nature of our wrongs.

Reluctance to continue with step five can be complicated. We might feel embarrassed about confessing to stupid behaviour or frightened that we will become open to manipulation. When we examine our reluctance honestly, a common reason for not wanting to continue is the belief that until we admit to our defects we can carry on enjoying whatever they give us.

Admitted to God, to ourselves and to another human being…

We might cynically claim that if God is "all-knowing" then he is already aware of everything and so we don't need to do this step. People down through the ages have kicked against their spiritual development with this excuse and we are no different. An omnipotent Higher Power may know about our defects, but it is now time for us to acknowledge them. There are common phrases like "skeletons in the closet" or "bottling things up" and more clinical terms such as suppression or repression to describe these hidden secrets. Whatever we call them, acknowledging our defects and understanding the pain they create is essential to a healthy way of life. One of the best ways to start to "own" these issues is to talk openly about them with somebody else.

Who should I talk to

When the original members created the Big Book, there wasn't the "luxury" of so many meetings and sober alcoholics. The hope was that people would be able to use the instructions in the Big Book to create their own local infrastructure. They offered a number of suggestions about sharing a step four; any trusted person, a doctor or a spiritual leader, it even suggests that we could choose a complete stranger.

For people not working through a clinical recovery program, the idea of taking a three-hour appointment with a doctor is probably out of the question. Whether this is viable depends upon how much our doctor is willing to become involved in our recovery.

A spiritual leader would almost certainly be willing to give the time to listen and this could be the correct thing to do if we are already part of an organised religion. Even for those of us without any religious affiliation there seems to be a strange attraction in talking to a "man of the cloth". Films and television create the impression that we "ought" to return to the church when we are trying to put our life straight. Remember the earlier warning, that if we become involved, we should be careful not to confuse the program and religion. They should remain separate activities within our life.

If we tried the complete stranger method, it is questionable that we would be able to stay honest about our character defects without manipulating the truth to present ourselves in the best light. The honest statement born in our mind can twist into justification by the time it leaves our mouth. We explain our side of a situation to get a response like, "They got what they deserved" or "I would have done just the same". This is human, not alcoholic behaviour. We prefer being blameless and wronged to scheming and flawed, but vindication is of no value to a step five. We are looking to honestly acknowledge our actions, not justify them, a complete stranger may listen, but it is questionable if it would work.

Today, most of us choose to share step five with our sponsor. By this stage, they should have a good understanding of us and be able to challenge as appropriate, but there can be reasons why our sponsor isn't the correct choice. The emotions created by talking about our intimate secrets are certainly a prime example of when "cross sex" sponsorship is difficult. If we have un-resolved criminal behaviour to disclose, these might be more correctly addressed outside the fellowship. Within AA, there are murderers, rapists and thieves with issues that require careful handling. Whilst a sponsor will be a loyal and close-lipped friend, they aren't priests, or trained in hearing confession. They aren't professionally bound by a code of silence. They are ex-drunks who are trying their best to stay sober. If there is an on-going concern such as child abuse, it is correct that our sponsor should challenge this and if required make the relevant authorities aware of the issue.

...the exact nature of our wrongs

The word "exact" means that we have to make sure that we can share our step four as honestly as possible. The choice of the other person and the location has a great bearing upon our ability to achieve this.

We probably shouldn't attempt step five in a public place, such as a restaurant or coffee bar. Many who proclaim that they never show emotion find themselves in tears at some point during their fifth step. It is hard to conceive of honestly sharing our innermost secrets whilst fearing that the couple at the next table are eavesdropping or that the waiter cleaning the table is laughing at our tears. Whilst we can do step five in a steamed up car in a lay-by, it is normal to do it in surroundings that are more comfortable. We possibly think that our home is suitable, but it isn't if we have family around. Partners can overhear, or children need feeding. This will probably be one of the most memorable events of our recovery. It is an extremely powerful experience and an important stage in our development. As such, it is worthy of some forethought and planning, we don't want any fear or interruption to hinder us.

It is also worth considering that we will take a few hours to uncover all of the issues we have become aware of and so we need to allow sufficient time and probably a plentiful supply of tea or coffee to keep both people going.

We need to be confident that we are revealing the untainted truth about ourselves and we can make sure that we stay honest by returning to the framework of our fourth step and the major headings, Pride, Greed and Lust etc. The person we share our step with can gently guide us, but they are not there to make judgement upon what they hear. They are providing our Higher Power with a set of ears to listen to our honest appraisal of our character defects.

There isn't a precise "how" to completing the step, the person, place and timing all contribute, but the most important factor is that we are willing to "see it through". Some people feel clumsy with written notes, or have reading difficulties. In doing our fourth step we have spent sufficient time investigating our moral defects to know them off by heart. It is perfectly acceptable to work from memory if we are confident that we are not deliberately holding anything back.

Other people find that working through their written notes gives them comfort and support. By using our fourth step notes, we can be certain that we have covered the topics we explored and identified as defective. We may prefer to prepare a short "crib card" of helpful one-word prompts to guide us and ensure that we don't forget anything.

Why am I doing this?

We rarely understand a step until we have completed it. Sharing these hidden secrets with another person often removes the embarrassment from them. We sometimes start to share incidents from our fourth step in open meetings and memories that once horrified us are now merely facts without any shame attached. This will not be true for all of it and some parts will remain confidential for the rest of our lives.

One of the principles of this step is ego-deflation. Creating the impression that we are infallible and maintaining an overbearing belief in our own importance is essential to most of us. Strangely, we can often mask our bloated ego behind a demeanour of inferiority. This means that a more correct term for the experience might be ego-rightsizing.

Some people describe the effect of doing their step five as orgasmic, possibly this is why they are tempted to do multiple step fives! However, we aren't doing the step for reasons of exhilaration and shouldn't be disappointed if this is not the case. If we are confident that we have exposed a complete moral inventory to ourselves, another person and to God, we can humbly recognise we have taken a huge step towards a new life.

And finally...

By the end of steps four and five, we should have a clear understanding of our defects and a list of examples of where they led us into harming people. This list will support us when we get to step eight.

There are suggestions of what we should do with our step four at this stage. Some suggest a ceremonial burning to display the end of that phase of our lives. Others favour keeping it for future reference to see how we change in years to come. Remember that if we do keep it, to put it somewhere that it will remain hidden. Life moves on and it can be embarrassing if somebody unexpectedly finds it.

Summary

- Are we confident that there is no incident hidden in our past that we have decided never to expose?

- Have we examined with rigorous honesty our involvement in any situation where somebody was hurt?

If we hesitate about answering yes to these questions, we are not yet ready to continue.

Step Six

The Bechers Brook of the program is crossed and we
expect a simple flat gallop for the finish line. The
instructions in the Big Book suggest that we immediately
complete steps six and seven. If we read these in the
Twelve Steps and Twelve Traditions, it describes step six
as the step that sorts out the men from the boys, implying
that we will now start to take responsibility for our actions
and our lives.

Why would the Big Book suggest we embark upon such
an important phase with seemingly undue haste?

The reason is one of timing. Steps four and five broke
through the shell of justification covering our defects
leaving them exposed and painful. If we allow it to heal
over, we will rationalise our old feelings and discover that
we are reluctant to change.

*Were entirely ready to have God remove all these defects of
character*

Were entirely ready...

If we identify something about ourselves that we accept as
a defect, why would we not be ready to have it removed?
There tends to be an intermingled set of justifications
preventing us from acting:

- Convention suggests that something is a defect, but
  we don't agree.

- Although through steps four and five we accept that
  our behaviour conflicts with "spiritual growth", we
  feel we still "need it" and therefore decide to
  consider doing something about it at a later time.

- We know that our behaviour is wrong, but we think that it is too much a part of us to give it up.

When we first stop drinking, we declare that we are willing to do anything to get sober. We see the fact that we were "willing" to stop drinking and change things that were about to kill us as proof of this. We are wrong. We hit a rock bottom and could see our destructive obsession for what it was, a choice between drink and death. Even then, we required help to change and have our obsession removed.

This is the first time we have a real choice. We can keep the defect and remain in our comfort zone, or change and stray into the unknown. Most of us initially choose to keep our defects and don't perceive them to be a direct threat to our sobriety. We possibly listen to "wiser" voices, but don't hear what they are saying. We bump into a brick wall and feel it is unacceptable for us to change. Strongly held convictions and statements like, "I could never forgive…" highlight these defects. For example, we can see that it is wrong to wish somebody harm, but circumstances assure us that this is the only correct option.

If we allow it to, the monkey on our shoulder will use these convictions as a reason to abandon the program, phrases like "they don't understand", will become part of our thinking. As we hesitate, the monkey will suggest that we need to go and talk to our friends who "really know us" rather than the new friends who seem to be guiding us along uncomfortable paths. By doing this, we will easily find somebody who will help us to justify our feelings.

The monkey is willing to fight to keep the pleasant home it has found. If it manages to trick us into justifying why we don't need to change, we remain trapped in a life of misery and confusion.

Financial pressures and debt

It is common to feel that becoming "too honest" endangers our earning capacity. Alcoholism has a voracious appetite for money and when we stop drinking, we often face large amounts of debt, even if it is manageable, the fear of financial insecurity can overwhelm us and poison our thinking.

In some industries, there are forms of "acknowledged" dishonesty, shop-workers can consider "dipping the till" to be an acceptable way to subsidise their wage and people claiming expenses can adjust the details in their favour. Others earn their living in a criminal or dubious way and cannot find an honest job to provide the same levels of reward. We argue that we will stop behaving this way at some time in the future, but believe it to be the only way to clear our outstanding debts and achieve sobriety.

Distorted self-awareness

In addition to the more obvious defects indicated by strongly held convictions and fears, there are more subtle forms. These are the defects we consider characteristics of our personality. We possibly think we can work longer and harder than anybody else can, or we enjoy our "forthright" reputation. It could be that we don't trust anybody else to prepare the meals for a dependent relative. We see these as assets and an important of part us, they are "who we are" and without them, we would become the hole in the doughnut.

In the case of the loving daughter who has shouldered the responsibility of looking after her elderly parents. Other family members could assist, but the alcoholic will frequently take control and occupy the centre stage. Inevitably, the alcoholic comes to feel that they have taken on too much and they hope or demand that others take some of the burden. If no help is forthcoming, they descend further into bitterness, complaining of the injustice of their position. If others do try to help, the alcoholic will immediately find fault in what they do and start trying to control them. Finally, they make the decision that nobody else is competent at the task and they snatch it back.

This is an example of behaviour drifting. The actions were acceptable under exceptional circumstances, but unacceptable in the long term. The drift is gradual and because we are suffering from an illness that blinds us to our behaviour, we sometimes need help to recognise it. By persisting in our own infallibility, we end up crippled by the weight of tasks we have gathered to ourselves.

Fear is certainly part of the motivation in such a situation, we want to ensure that things function correctly, but pride is a much stronger part of it. Looked at from a different point of view we are stealing the happiness from family life for our own selfish reasons. Whilst we feel comfortable in our position of control, our demands can be overbearing. We push others to the point where they react badly and we see their aggressive reaction as proof that they don't value us.

When our behaviour is the cause of unnecessary distress to other people, we have to consider it a defect. An indication that there is a problem is if we are defending our actions by claiming that people must accept us the way we are. Unnecessary distress could be, selectively enforcing "rules" upon some people, whilst ignoring them for others, just because we feel like it. It might be spoiling somebody else's pleasure, for a laugh or for spite. These are possibly frivolous examples, but the key telltale is that people are hurt who would not have expected us to be the cause of their pain.

Some of us work in senior roles and have to make decisions that affect people. As we recover from alcoholism, our role can present us with confusing dilemmas. If for sound business reasons we have to dismiss somebody, we should have the strength and courage to carry out our duty. Under these circumstances, we are not causing unnecessary distress, but acting in a responsible manner.

…to have God remove…

The step does not say that we removed them. It says that we _were entirely ready to have God remove them_. We have already had the first of our major defects lifted by the removal of the urge to drink destructively. We can see that "something" outside of us achieved this. The next defect is our need for control and self-determination. We will change our old unacceptable behaviour by _unreservedly_ accepting outside influence on how our life is going to change.

…all of these defects of character

Where the first part of the program involved looking at our past behaviour to prove where our self-will had put us. We are now going to look at how we act and behave today. Even more than this, we are going to accept that our behaviour is flawed and believe that we can change.

We can usually see the benefits of a sober life, but we want these benefits without effort and discomfort, unfortunately this is not what the program offers. It offers a life that becomes better than our drinking life, but this is conditional; expecting things to improve without allowing change is exactly like expecting to row across a lake whilst the boat remains tethered to the dock. We can put as much effort into rowing as we want, but we will just get tired and disheartened at our lack of progress.

Drilling through these defects

To remove the defects that are hindering our progress we can question ourselves and try to identify in what way these defects really contribute to a peaceful life? If our justifications quickly descend into worn out statements like "somebody has to do something", "the pope could solve the problem of famine from the coffers of the Vatican" then we are probably ranting in an egotistical manner. Our rant usually isn't contributing anything. If we feel that it is, then we should drill through the first statement and examine it further. Are we really the "somebody" who can achieve anything? Can we really change the behaviour of an institution like the church?

We can repeatedly apply honest appraisal to penetrate these platitudes and reach the core, which is that our strongly held belief adds nothing to anybody's life, certainly not ours.

We can pursue this "drilling through" on any defect that seems to be worth hanging on to. There are examples in AA of people forgiving the unforgivable. They come to terms with the violent death of a loved one, or have been able to let go of the feelings resulting from the rape of a young daughter. When the emotional surface of the defect is penetrated and the value looked for, we rarely find anything worth keeping. If we think that there is value, then we should talk to our sponsor and discuss these feelings in detail.

There may be defects that seem impossible to address "yet", but we can work towards the willingness to have them removed. This is not an excuse to procrastinate indefinitely, but a viable route forwards.

In our early days in AA, we might have come to hate the word "yet". Whenever we said something along the lines of "I have not been in prison…" somebody would add – yet, emphasising the downward spiral waiting for us if we returned to drinking. Now it comes into play in a positive way, we are not willing – yet, but we can work towards it. The willingness to become willing allows us to consider changing in order to recover.

What happens if we remain unwilling to have a defect removed?

Although the step only requires a willingness to have the defect removed, this doesn't mean that we take no responsibility for our actions.

As a child, I loved to play in the garden. I would be swinging from the tree and see my mother start to prepare the car to go to the shops. I knew what was coming- I was going to have my hair brushed and have to go with her. I always played out the tantrum of how unfair she was being. She always responded by saying, "kicking and screaming, or happy and smiling, you are coming to the shops – now choose."

This also describes what happens for us when we stubbornly refuse to make progress with removing our defects. Our Higher Power allows chaos to build until we accept that we need to change.

Does this seem a bit too weird? This is the first time we have suggested that the Higher Power is not just a concept, but takes actions within our lives.

I sometimes see myself as Elmer Fudd in the cartoons (copyright

Warner Brothers, little man, bald head, hates wabbits) and I imagine myself proceeding slowly down a darkening tunnel. As I walk, I see sign after sign, "Don't go this way", "Danger – This means YOU". Do I pay attention? Not a bit, I have my entire being focused upon shooting that darned wabbitt. Finally, in the near black gloom I sit down on a convenient box and strike a match. All the onlookers can see that the box says "DYNAMITE," but I sit there and drop the match...

If we see and act upon the sensible notices and warnings that life shows us, we live with the minimum of pain. Exactly as depicted in the cartoon, the strength of the warnings increases as we continue to ignore them. Charred and blinking we realise the mess we are in and finally become willing to do something. We are not made to suffer without cause, or for some "deeper purpose," it is just our Higher Power waiting for us to pay attention.

Any time we feel like we are cornered, having to justify our actions, we are probably embarking on yet another Fudd-like descent down a dark tunnel. This is invariably true if our actions bring us into conflict with people or acceptable behaviour. When our actions start to require secrecy, or when guilt is creeping in, then we have identified a defect. Having identified it, can we develop the willingness to have it removed?

Summary

To maintain the determination to carry on with this, we must come back to the primary purpose of why we are doing the program. We are not trying to become "better people," we are doing this to get well. We are currently following a path and the signpost says ALL of these defects, not just those we choose. Even if we cannot see the reason for removing them, they have to go. We certainly don't lose any portion of our personality that makes us "us". As promised, we lose the defects.

- Are we holding onto anything that could be directly or indirectly the cause harm to other people?

- Do we feel that a level of dishonesty is acceptable?

If we cannot answer no to these questions, we should look for help before we proceed. Without doing so, it is pointless trying to go much further. These defects will taint our progress, we won't achieve a contented sobriety and we will probably drink again.

Communicating with a higher power

This short section comes before step seven for a reason. The seventh step instructs us to ask God to remove all our shortcomings and if we reject the idea of a God, we are at the kind of impasse that leads to giving up on the program.

If our Higher Power is of the spiritual variety, we probably feel that prayer is the correct way to communicate, but we should almost certainly wait until after we have reached step eleven before depending upon this as a normal method of communicating with our Higher Power.

This is not to suggest that prayer is wrong, but we often try to adopt an answer without fully understanding the implications of what we are doing. Once we have reached our sixth step, our enthusiasm for the program and spiritual living leaves us open to a different style of attack from the monkey. We are eager to progress and we think that asking for guidance on how to pray is like asking how to fall off a log, a voice says, "How hard can it be?" We need to tread carefully, within an organised religion, somebody with experience helps novices to avoid pitfalls by leading the prayer and it is too easy for us to become confused when we approach this on our own.

When we start to use prayer and meditation, we are looking to become a radio receiver capable of detecting the messages sent by our Higher Power. Just like radio waves, these are undetectable unless we have sensitive equipment that we know how to use. Unfortunately, the monkey is sitting in a taxicab parked nearby and can transmit so strongly that it overpowers any other signal. Currently, it is too easy for the monkey to supplant the messages from our Higher Power with messages of its own. The thoughts can seem logical and well reasoned, but when we look at them rationally, they prove to be the illness in disguise. Thoughts like, "If God doesn't want me to make that call tomorrow I will find that the telephone is not working" or "If I am not meant to sell my car it will be stolen" are examples of the monkey subverting rational thinking.

The guidance for step eleven is to "ask for knowledge of God's will for us and the power to carry it out", but this does not infer that all messages from our Higher Power will travel through the ether. It can be a request to guide us towards people to talk to and the humility to discuss our problems honestly. If our GOD (Group Of Drunks) is the fellowship of AA, they are sitting and waiting to help. The only obstacle is our pride. Regardless of the nature of our chosen Higher Power, it is possible to communicate directly and openly. Although we might have wished for something more fantastical than this, once again the answer is simply talking to people.

Those with a "spiritual" higher power can feel challenged by the suggestion that they shouldn't rely on prayer, but if we consider it with an open mind, by talking and listening we give our higher power a mouth, not just at meetings, but on a one to one basis, face to face or on the phone.

Late one night, the phone rang. It was somebody from the meeting I didn't know much about. He said he was feeling lost and uncertain about his sobriety. We chatted for a few minutes and then I heard myself say, "How long have you been having an affair?" It came out of my mouth, but I have no idea where the statement came from. The silence at the end of the line told me that we were treading upon uncertain ground. He hesitated and then started to pour out a tale of living with deception and lies for the last few months. Unable to share honestly, his sobriety was failing, but he hadn't looked at it. That simple enquiry changed his life. I am amazed each time I think of this. I hadn't known anything about him, but somehow I had asked the right question at the right time.

We find that examples like this happen frequently and talking to trusted friends is a positive method of communicating with our Higher Power. If this feels too much like we are straying into unacceptably "woolly" god territory, it isn't. We should consider that the humanistic branches of counselling have proved that there are therapeutic effects whenever two people are in psychological contact in a safe and trusting environment. We achieve this scientifically proven environment whenever we talk to other people within AA, providing we stay within the framework of experience, strength, and hope.

For this communication to work three things must be in place:

- We have to be honest about our feelings, actions and intentions.

- The other person must be able to listen and provide valid feedback.

Most importantly:

- We have to listen to the feedback, and be willing to change from our current course.

Just as the mask in a masquerade ball disguises our identity, an emotional mask attempts to disguise our true emotions. Wearing emotional masks is part of normal life. We sometimes want to make people think well of us or to intimidate them, at other times it is to hide our fears or suppress our anger. A mask helps us get on with people and it is unrealistic to expect to live without adopting one. However, it is a good idea to make a mental check and clear away our masks when we talk with another member of AA. We should be willing to expose our plans, actions and emotions honestly, regardless of how we feel about doing so. We are masters of justification and can easily lead other people towards our chosen answer.

People within AA will give us their time and attention, they are not merely nodding their heads in agreement, as our confidantes of old might have, but are considering carefully what we have said to them. They listen and often when we least expect or desire it, question our motives, explaining that either they or a close friend has ended up in trouble by doing what we are suggesting.

We not only have to listen to what the other person has to say, we also have to be willing to act upon it. They can reveal things that we had not thought of, throwing our preferred path into question, leaving us with a number of choices. We can go and ask somebody else's opinion, we can ignore them and continue with what we are currently planning or we can believe the person we have asked and change our plan.

There is no "correct" answer in this situation, but we soon find that it is pointless and potentially dangerous to "poll" opinion on a defect. If we ask enough people about something, we will eventually find somebody who agrees with us. If we choose to ignore all advice and carry on anyway we need to be on extremely sure ground because if somebody we trust challenges our behaviour with coherent reasons, they are probably right.

Summary:

By staying close to people who have trodden the path, we allow our chosen higher power to guide us without thunderbolts or burning bushes.

Step Seven

It seems odd that although we are repeatedly told that each step is individual and must be approached in its own right, we are then confronted by the fact that they are discussed as rhyming couplets, four and five, six and seven, eight and nine, none more so than the "hidden steps," six and seven. They lie nestled, hidden, between the four big "action" steps and possibly because they don't ask us to do something tangible we feel they are merely padding, placed to provide a breather between the obvious hurdles surrounding them. This isn't true. Six and Seven free us of the shackles of our past, allowing us to enjoy the sunlight of the new life that is on offer.

We have acknowledged our defects in painstaking detail through steps four and five, but these defects will remain active and troublesome until we take specific action to have them removed. Six and Seven are "used" together, because once we are ready to have a defect removed, it seems only logical to move onto the step that enables this to happen.

Humbly asked Him to remove our shortcomings.

Humbly...

Humility as a concept is frequently misunderstood, possibly through association with people like Uriah Heep in Dickens, claiming to be "ever so 'umble" whilst in reality being scheming and arrogant. The word reeks of religion and Sunday school lessons. We conjure visions of false humility and we reject the concept before considering the real implications.

There is the well-worn cliché, "If you realise you have humility – you just lost it." By this simple phrase, we prevent discussion of what is a cornerstone of the program. It is easier to discuss sexual perversion in a meeting than to discuss humility in a meaningful way. If we encounter somebody quoting this cliché, we should question what the person is saying. They might believe that repeating "clever sayings" like a parrot makes them appear wise, or they could have identified that we are proud of our humility. Depending upon which is true, give them a cracker or thank them. The monkey on our shoulder must be splitting his sides with laughter each time he tricks somebody into quoting it to us. Thanks to such a subtle trap, we find ourselves unable to ask people for help at a point when we desperately need it.

As with so many clichés, it is valid when used within context. We would certainly need our bubble bursting if we suggested that we had achieved the humility of St. Francis, but we can recognise when our behaviour is acceptable and we can certainly aspire to improve. The problem is how can we improve our humility without discussion?

Humility is about modestly acknowledging our true worth to society and not about vainly hoping to atone for our past behaviour by pretending to be a doormat. Through the program, we provide an effective framework to constrain our over-active ego and achieve an acceptable level of humility.

...asked Him...

A memory that always stays with me is standing in the shower, naked and covered in soap. I was beating my fist on the wall demanding that God took some action and did it now! Ironically, I was asking to have my irrational anger removed. Suddenly, I saw a snapshot of this scene as if from outside of myself, giving me the gift of seeing the arrogance in my behaviour and showing me how others see me. I had to laugh at the futility of this soapy, beached whale threatening violence against the power I had claimed to acknowledge as greater than myself. Thankfully, this vision and laughter meant that I took another step towards understanding humility.

Regardless of the form of our chosen Higher Power, it isn't a genie capable of fulfilling unreasonable requests and a first step towards accepting spirituality is recognising how to ask for help. Help is always available, but rarely in the form that we anticipate.

If our Higher Power is the group and we don't approach it with humility, we will almost certainly receive rapid and tangible feedback. If we try to demand that the meeting answers our personal need to get sober, we will certainly get a response. The result of such a demand is usually a dose of "tough love", directing us into looking at our approach and attitude. Whilst this will initially sting our pride, we hopefully recover and come to thank the group for their help and honesty.

...To remove our shortcomings

Once we understand how our Higher Power communicates, as well as starting to live with humility, we are equipped to work on the defects. As one defect falls another seems to become apparent. We can look on these as crops or phases. The first crop of defects is easy to identify, as time passes other defects of the "part of me" category become apparent.

Our cycle of progress becomes self-supporting as we recognise that by changing our way of thinking - our emotions and behaviour also change. We become aware that change is possible. We see that we don't lose anything that forms the real "us", but we do lose the liabilities. As we acknowledge this, we become more willing to accept that change can be a good thing. Finally, we discover that we are progressing towards a faith. We have not had to accept faith blindly, but we know that our life is improving and we are not solely responsible.

We are a set of garden shears lost at the back of the shed. They are now blunt with the central pivot screw loose. The Gardener needs them for a specific job and regrets losing them. As a set of shears, we have no concept of our purpose, but the gardener does. Once retrieved, he will tighten the screw, sharpen the blades and return us into service. By removing the defects, we can fulfil our role.

It is our responsibility to identify the defects and ask to have them removed. It is also our responsibility to try to ensure that these defects do not come back. It generally appears to be true that our Higher Power doesn't intervene unless either we ask, or we blindly head too far into danger. It certainly doesn't work based on stating, "I am full of defects, you know what they are, remove them". We have to return to our fourth step list and specifically identify them.

Practice the opposite

The world's major religions (Christianity, Islam, Hindu, Sikh, Buddhism and Judaism) all suggest Pride, Lust, Anger and Greed as damaging behaviour. There is a similar consensus about the way to avoid them by the conscious practice of the opposite. They all identify Charity, Humility and Compassion as positive character traits that we should aspire to have in our lives. It would seem impossible to damage people through lustful or angry behaviour if we viewed them with compassion. The way to acquire such virtues is the subject of many thousands of inspirational pages, but the essence is the same, quoted in no specific order:

- To treat others as we would wish to be treated

- To respect other people and humbly aspire to be worthy of their respect

- To seek to understand rather than to be understood

Keeping a change in place

Many notice a strange phenomenon that occurs as soon as we make the decision to address a defect, we are immediately overwhelmed with a feeling of euphoria and peace. Our determination to change can weaken. The pain created by the defect seems to lift and the idea of addressing the problem drifts completely out of our consciousness.

Why this occurs is difficult to explain, unless we attribute the monkey on our shoulder with the intelligence to be devious. By whispering warm and pleasant thoughts, the illness defends against us reducing its influence. This seems difficult to accept, but we all experience this during our recovery.

My relationship with my wife was bad and I started to enjoy chatting with one of the women at the meeting. When we decided to travel to meetings together the sexual tension grew. I felt alive. It had been a long time since I had enjoyed laughter and infatuation. Things seemed perfect, we both agreed that we would just have fun and that neither of us wanted more. My stomach dropped when I got the message that she wanted us to set up home together. The fun in our relationship switched to fear and recrimination. Each time my wife answered the phone I thought she was about to be told that I was living a lie.

I went to my sponsor and told him. We agreed that I had to

break off all contact – immediately. I left his house and headed
for my girlfriends home. I arrived and everything seemed to have
changed. She was happy and alive. We laughed and as we
tumbled, the idea of ending things faded. I thought, "Why on
earth should I change this?"

Defects always rise again. They come back, the pain is
more intense and this allows the monkey to play another
trick. Regardless of the fact that we didn't actually follow
our original plan, we think that we did. We recall that we
have been in this position before and that we took action
to remove the defect. Believing the program failed we look
outside for an answer.

With practice, we learn to expect this burst of euphoria
and know that we must not be distracted. As we proceed
with the change, the euphoria dissolves and life becomes
dismal, possibly even unbearable. The degree the monkey
fights against a change has a direct relationship to the
benefit that is waiting for us.

Summary:

We will never remove all of our defects and these are life
long exercises. Armed with the belief that it works and
that life gets better each time we work to remove a defect
through the practice of step six and seven, it actually
becomes a pleasure. With each character defect we
remove, we put another brick into place in the fabric of the
new life we are building.

•   Can I identify the opposite of my defect?

•   Have I a clear way to communicate with my higher
     power?

Defect Dogs

Imagine living in a small town where every day we need to journey from one side to the other. There are many possible routes, shortest, fastest, boring, or pleasant. We want to use the quickest, but the problem is that a large vicious dog lives on this route. Each time we go along it, the dog appears snarling and snapping at us.

We try to complain about the owner, but when we enquire, we find that most people think the dog belongs to us and they wish we would control it because it is making their lives hell. Our first reaction might be that we will arm ourselves and give it such a thrashing that it won't come near us again. Anybody who has encountered powerful dogs knows that this is a hopeless idea. Once the dog has started to attack, it is uncontrollable and deadly beyond any defence we can muster. We cannot fight, kill or control it. The only option is avoiding it. We may feel that we are running away from a problem that we should be able to face, but eventually we come to see that this is the only answer.

Avoiding the dog means becoming willing to change our normal life and go a different way. This change will mean that we have to take a bit more time and find our way around parts of the town that we have not visited before.

The dog is a representation of our worst defects and the monkey often brings this other animal into our life. When we were drinking, we spent so much time with the dog strutting at our heels that everybody assumed it was ours. Strangely in our drinking days we either didn't know it was there or we laughed at how it intimidated the people we met.

Those of us who have experienced uncontrollable anger

know this feeling well. We encounter something that triggers our violent reaction and our emotions flare out of control leaving us a bystander in the torrent of verbal and physical abuse we hurl, but the dog is not just a representation of anger. Once unleashed, any of the major defects can take over and leave us with little control.

A friend had commented that I was always late for the start of the meeting. I was determined to change this and so I volunteered to bring the milk and tea. I was sure this would focus my mind.

I found that each week just before I left the house, somebody in the family would desperately need my attention. Each week one of my children needed me. Billy had forgotten to pick up the children's homework or Betty was leaving her husband. I had to drive across town to solve their problems and then feel guilty that I had let the meeting down.

Sometimes I would try and put the meeting first, but then I felt I was letting my family down. Regardless of my choice, I ended up feeling guilty. I don't know if I will ever get it fully under control, but I know that unless I keep focused on my right to have some time for myself I end up battered by my desire to help. It would be nice if they would stop having their problems, but I am the only person I can change and so that is what I am doing. One day at a time, I try not to carry my entire family.

It is not easy to keep the dog out of our lives. It has been a part of us for longer than we can remember and to expect it simply to cease to exist is unrealistic. We are changing the way we live and this change does not always feel natural or normal. We have pushed the dog away. It is gone, but prowls close by, waiting for a chance to take its place at our heels again.

Every day of our life, we have to make the decision to use the more scenic route rather than risk awakening the dog.

Step Eight

We are now at what we thought was the second major hurdle of the program, but if we completely ignore the implications of step nine, step eight becomes quite easy.

Made a list of all persons we had harmed and became willing to make amends to them all.

This demonstrates the wonderful subtlety of the building nature of the program. In step four, we identified a defect in our behaviour. In step five, we acknowledged the defect to another person (and our Higher Power). In step six, we became willing to have it removed. In step seven, we asked our Higher Power to remove it. We should be convinced that the defect now has no place in our new life. We are not simply clearing away the debris of our old existence. We are reviewing our actions in a way that highlights our previous conduct. By taking ownership of our past behaviour, we are defining our own moral guidelines. Although we have never been good at living by rules defined by others, we should be able to live by a set that we define for ourselves.

By breaking the step down into three specific phrases, we can examine it in detail and see that each part in itself is easy. It says nothing about taking any action towards these people, it merely involves being honest with ourselves about how we have affected them.

Made a list...

We undertook a large part of this during step four and we are now going to build upon that earlier work. Our list will typically have three columns, names, the harm we feel we have done, and the amends we feel are due. Nothing more complicated than a pen and paper is required.

We know the behaviours and defects we identified and we start from this. Major headings are useful to trigger memories, Sex, Work, Resentment, Jealousy and Family are good starting points. We often punished people who loved us and we can examine our relationship with every close member of our family: spouse, children, siblings and parents. There are usually many amends to make amongst our loved ones and the thought of trying to make them drives home the burden of guilt. We continually need to revisit the statement that we were sick and suffering from an illness.

During the creation of this list, it can be useful to return to step four and widen our thinking. By doing this we can identify similar incidents and situations. Through practicing self-examination, we illuminate many more dark corners. It is a surprise how far back in our lives we can go and still see damaging behaviour, certainly farther back than we previously thought drink had adversely affected our conduct.

...Of all persons we had harmed...

Persons, not institutions, we can rarely claim the Local Hospital was offended by our actions. If we can identify a particular nurse, recall a specific incident and suggest a meaningful amend, then this person belongs on the list.

We need to be aware of the nature of the harm; we do harm when we try to impose our will on another, causing pain and distress through thoughtless or malicious action. This occurs when we believe other people don't deserve the same consideration or compassion we would expect for ourselves.

The illness of alcoholism involves much more than drinking. Drunk or sober, alcoholics have a tendency to damage people. Sometimes it is unintentional, like a boisterous large child hurting other children in a playgroup. At other times, it is a more calculated harm, varying between great extremes, from murder, rape, and physical abuse through to petty jealousy and gossip. We sometimes damage people with wholly good intentions, by being over-protective of them instead of allowing them to make their own mistakes.

Before going much farther, it is useful to reflect upon this. The anguish caused by murder or rape can be easily imagined, but few of us have directly experienced it, whereas many of us have suffered from malicious gossip at some stage in our life. We judge based upon our own experience, feeling that anything we have been able to survive is acceptable for other people. Unfortunately, this is not true and has no bearing upon the harm that we caused. We cannot judge how badly we hurt somebody; anybody we harmed should be on the list.

...and became willing to make amends to them all

It doesn't suggest how or when we shall take any action, but specifically says, ALL and became willing. It is perfectly normal to add somebody to the list, but as we are writing to think, "I will never do this". The step is in two parts to help guard against only adding people when we are willing to make amends. There are a few reasons why we would not want to include somebody on our list.

Fear, is often present, we fear the retribution they will unleash, or imagine that it is too humiliating to face them. They can still go on the list. This is why this step is separate from the actual act of making amends.

Recognising these fears is a healthy part of the step.

Justification, at the suggestion that we have done wrong we normally start to justify why we were forced into an unavoidable situation. To acknowledge that we intentionally harmed people is accepting that we are capable of bullying, sadistic, self-centred or dishonest behaviour.

Unwilling, to acknowledge the harm we have done because we believe the harm they did to us is "unforgivable" and so we are unwilling to contemplate ever being in contact with the person again. The simple fact is that if we are blameless and we are entirely the victim then this person has no place on our list. If we have played a part in harming somebody, regardless of their role then we have to look at how we can become willing to make amends to them.

Forgiving is frequently an obstacle. The phrase "I will never forgive…" previously suggested as heralding a difficult defect is with us again. There is a well-known saying *"to err is human, to forgive divine"* and it is safe to say that most people have a problem with the concept of forgiveness. Unfortunately, where others are able to, we cannot hide behind platitudes. Later, in step nine, we may hope for forgiveness, but part of step eight is that we have to learn ways to become willing to forgive other people (and ourselves).

Do not look for too much advice

Frequently the monkey suggests that we need to go and discuss our actions with somebody present at an incident. The people we turn to are biased in our favour and may collude with us to mitigate what occurred. They don't understand our recovery program and will not want to consider us humbling ourselves in front of our common enemy. By discussing our actions with people outside of AA, it is easy to get the reaction that we want – "they got what they deserved", giving us the freedom to cross a name off the list

How many people should be on our list? Asking other people how many people were on their list is like asking how much somebody earns, rarely polite and often not answered. It is a deeply personal issue, but extremely confusing for most of us. A practising alcoholic will have stood on the toes of hundreds of people in the crowd, how do we ascertain if we should include them on the list?

We may never find the shop assistant we verbally abused, but if their face pushes out from "the crowd" and we remember the incident, we should write them down, it is important to acknowledge the repetition of our actions.

A character defect I discovered was that I liked "nice things". When I visited people's homes, I looked with envy at their possessions and occasionally small objects came home with me. I felt that I deserved them and that my friend would want me to be happy.

Obviously, I eventually abused all of my friendships and I was terrified of facing them. I continually conjured the scene, their returned ornaments, trinkets, tins of salmon, and bottles of wine spread on the table whilst they scornfully told me what they thought of me, expelling me from their homes and their lives forever.

A common temptation is to avoid the painful situations by "swamping" the list with trivia. We include people where there is no amend due because we know they will be forgiving and pat us on the back for our efforts.

To pare it down to revealing proportions we need to ask

specific questions, "What is the harm that was done?" and "What is the amend due?" If we don't have a clear answer to these questions, we are possibly padding the list.

Summary

We had felt that our past was a liability and that we needed to keep it locked away forever. Examining it in step eight, reveals that our past marks the path towards a life based upon moral guidelines that we agree to. Miraculously, the old structure is now being recycled to provide the building blocks of our new life.

•   Have we left anybody off the list for any reason?

This is the only check we need to carry out. Having six or six hundred people on our list is the correct number for us, providing we haven't deliberately omitted anybody.

Step Nine

The perfect journalistic story is ruled by the five sacred "W"s, What, Who, When, How and Why, these headings also provide a good framework to define step nine. The previous eight steps have been about changing our behaviour, feelings and demeanour by acceptance of concepts like fear, humility and pride. It is easy to practice the principles of the fellowship whilst we are at a meeting, but in this step, we are taking our new demeanour for a test drive and exhibiting it to people outside of our comfort zone.

Made direct amends to such people wherever possible, except when to do so would injure them or others.

WHAT are we going to do?

Made direct amends...

The statement is simple, made direct amends. For some people the amends required will be obvious, but we can be confident that a simple mumbling of sorry is insufficient. We should be willing to do whatever is required so that we are able to look these people in the eye without feeling shame and remorse.

WHO are we going to talk to?

... to such people...

We made our list in step eight and regardless of how many people are on it, we have to decide how to work through them.

Close family and friends who will welcome what we are

saying, these people are the ones who have stood by us beyond the point any human would have thought possible. They will have already witnessed a change in us and they will probably listen and readily forgive us.

Work colleagues and acquaintances, these people may prove surprisingly difficult to approach. They don't know us well, but we want to think they have a good opinion of us.

Damaged family and friends, these people, once close to us, now estranged, will be surprised and intrigued when we approach and ask to speak to them. They form the category that probably contains the highest number of the people we want to slot into the get out clause, *"except where to do so would injure them or others"*.

Virtual strangers, these are the people that we have no social relationship with. These can be senior managers through to people on the checkout at the supermarket.

WHEN are we going to do it?

The danger of getting the timing wrong

It is a mistake to leap into this activity before completing the first eight steps. We should do the steps in the correct order to fully understand and benefit from the process.

As soon as I started to get sober, I saw this step and thought that it was as an opportunity to say sorry. My soon to be ex-wife had seen and heard many Oscar winning performances and had finally gathered the strength to push me out of her life. I hoped that my "shiny new" remorse would fool her into accepting me back. She told me that although she understood what I was saying, she wanted to see action and change. I felt bitterly rejected because it had not worked out as I had expected it to.

The first thought that went through my mind was "I'll show her what she has made me do…" and I headed for a drink.

Whilst we are experiencing the pink cloud of the honeymoon period, telling people that we are complete idiots is another opportunity to become the centre of attention. It becomes much harder once we understand fully the implications of what we are doing and we have a better understanding of the effect our actions have on other people. If we leap in too early and our "amends" are accepted, we breathe a sigh of relief and fall back into old ways. If they reject us, we may consider that going back drinking will punish them and make them feel guilty for how they have treated us.

…except when to do so would injure them or others.

We have to work through the list and we often try to use a perceived risk of harm as an excuse not to do it. By honestly evaluating the situations and people involved and by discussing our proposed actions with our sponsor, we can start to clear away the debris from our past life.

Easy to approach, it is sensible to start with this group of people and get off to a good start. Although we are sitting with a close friend, we can find ourselves surprisingly tongue-tied.

Embarrassing to approach, having worked through the easier ones we will have developed a "technique" of calming our mind and introducing the reason we are doing this.

Painful to approach, this pain might be emotional or it could be financial. It can take some time to get to the stage where we can approach these people.

Too fearful to approach, there will be people we feel unable to approach. With this group, we sometimes have to start not from being willing to make amends to them, but work on becoming willing to be willing. This is not avoiding the issue, it is sometimes the best we can do. If we have such people on our list and we know that amends are due, we can allow time to pass and our emotions to mature to the point where we can speak to them. The experience of most of us is that the statement never is too final. The program and time treat the sting and pain of past memories, with help we grow up and change our view of people.

Unable to find, if it is impossible to find the person, then they must remain on our list, with the promise that if the means becomes available to locate them we will do so and make the appropriate amends.

Dead, doesn't always mean that we have fully lost the opportunity to make amends. It can be a fulfilling experience to stand by a memorial stone and apologise. If we cannot bring ourselves to offer a prayer for the dead, then we have to live in the knowledge that we had been willing to make amends.

Should not approach, our quest for rigorous honesty does not include apologising to the partner of our last affair, such acts of bravado and cruelty have no place in the "new us". Apologising to our lover, by saying that sickness was the basis of the "love affair" is probably a cruel and thoughtless act.

We have to be extremely careful if the situation we are going to create will risk losing our livelihood, we could be damaging our family with a grandiose gesture. Luring us into this style of thinking is one of the monkey's more subtle tricks. Financially crippled, "under the instructions of AA", we declare with righteous indignation that we destroyed our lives and were better off when we were drinking.

We must honestly consider a fear of suffering criminal violence. It can be too easy for people who do not know the party concerned to offer unfounded encouragement resulting in us becoming crippled or killed. If these are genuine fears, we are harming them by our amends. We can remain willing to make amends should the circumstances change.

By working through these categories, we are able to cross people off the list quite quickly and work down to the ones who are difficult or impossible to contact. As we become emotionally stronger, we can then approach those who are more difficult.

It is impossible to suggest a timescale for this step. If we have reached this stage of the program, we are becoming capable of making these decisions for ourselves.

HOW do we do it?

We should always approach people with humility. We know why we are doing this and what we think is a correct amends to offer, they don't and we should not expect them to. All of the steps are about changing our own behaviour. They are not about changing other people.

We need to be aware of the impact we can have on somebody, it is almost certainly inappropriate to discuss these issues whilst standing in line in the staff canteen. It is easy for us to become offhand about declaring ourselves to be alcoholic and working the program. For most people the word alcoholic conjures up images of ragged tramps on park benches.

If we make sure that the words *humble* and *sensitive* are in our minds as we approach somebody, we should be able to approach them correctly. We must also defend against switching to retaliation and justification if the person does not react as well as we had expected them to. They could take the opportunity to reveal issues that we had not even considered.

WHY are we doing this?

When this is complete - we are free from our past. Although the monkey will remain on our shoulder for the rest of our lives, we have now removed his ability to wound us with remorse and shame.

As we talk to the people on our list, they might suggest that we have reached this point through our own will power and efforts. It could be tempting to allow such a misconception to continue, but it is better to remain humble and acknowledge that our recovery comes from working the program. If they want to argue, allow them to believe what they choose as long as we don't believe it. We need to recognise that we have reached this point through the help of the fellowship and by the guidance and protection of our higher power.

Summary Questions

• Am I progressing through my list?

• Have I avoided anybody that I could approach?

Step Ten

Don't drink and don't die...

We are now free! We have addressed our old behaviour and if we have been practising each step of the program on a daily basis, we should be finding that life has improved. There are times when things don't go as well as we would wish – "living in reality" can be tough, but we shouldn't be involved in as many dramas as we used to be and when we are, we cope appropriately. We feel good and so it comes as a surprise when we hear "old-timers" proclaim that the best is yet to come.

Anybody who has children, or remembers being one, knows the anguished cry, "You don't understand". As a child, we cannot conceive of our parents suffering our distress. As we grow, we realise how childish our adolescent outbursts were. We come to understand that "being grown up" isn't a final position, but more like the rings in a tree trunk, a point in time from where we continue to grow and each year, life becomes progressively deeper and richer. Our ability to deal with problems continues to increase in line with our acceptance and practise of the program. Our life can improve to become better than our best times drinking, but it is essential to remember that the program grants a reprieve from the illness, not a cure. The monkey is waiting for the opportunity to regain control and tempt us back into old behaviour.

Continued to take personal inventory and when we were wrong promptly admitted it.

Our building work is complete and we are now living in our house. Anybody who has moved into a new home knows that there are various phases to go through. In the first few months, there is the "snagging" process. As time passes, the plaster cracks, doorframes settle and maintenance is required, a building is only fault free for a short period and there is always another problem waiting to emerge. We have reached the end of the house building analogy, but that doesn't mean that the work is over. It is actually just beginning as we move into our maintenance phase.

Continued to take personal inventory...

Most alcoholics have learned the hard way what happens to a living space that is not regularly cleaned and tidied. Housekeeping is usually something that we do a small amount of every day and attend to larger tasks on specific evenings or weekends. It would be rare if we didn't have a routine and we know that our life is unnecessarily uncomfortable if we don't keep up with it. Such as, we wash the dishes after each meal. If we don't stick to this, we end up with an unsightly pile of dirty dishes balanced precariously on the draining board. We know that it makes sense to do them every day, but sometimes we just don't want to...

Similarly, we know that we have to dust, clean the toilet, change the bedding etc. A routine makes it easier to achieve all of the jobs without forgetting anything.

In the case of inventory taking, it is common to repeat a complete inventory similar to the fourth step, although some prefer to do this by maintaining regular contact with their sponsor. In addition to this, we keep an eye on ourselves by establishing the habit of performing regular "quick inventory" checks.

A good time to take a quick inventory is just before we go to sleep. It can be part of a wind down routine. We can relax, review the day and see if we have allowed any of our regular defects to creep back into our lives. By now we should have abandoned being offended by idea's "borrowed" from a specific religion. The Christians talk of the seven deadly sins, Pride, Envy, Gluttony, Lust, Anger, Greed and Sloth. In broad terms, these describe categories of defects that are part of everybody's life. It might not be a good acronym by which to remember them, but PEGLAGS can work as an aide-memoir. By simply saying each word and looking at how we have acted during the day, we can form an idea of how we have behaved.

We should also evaluate what we have done well. In our earlier step four stock-take, we focused upon the negative parts of our inventory. We should now be able to acknowledge our good traits. Done with humility, this is acceptable and desirable as it encourages them to flourish.

At times our old way of thinking and behaving seems like that of another person. Most days we cannot comprehend how we hid upstairs listening to life downstairs and felt unable to face it, or how we always tried to control everybody. Inevitably, some parts of our old behaviour will creep back in.

<u>Anger</u>: Where others have the freedom to lose their temper without consequence, we no longer can. This doesn't mean that we don't lose our temper, but it means that we pay for it later. Irrational emotional outbursts leave us a trembling wreck for hours afterwards and so we try not to do it any more.

<u>Allowing the old life back in</u>: there is the temptation to get involved with friends and situations from our old life. Whilst not all old ties and connections need to be broken, we should examine our motives. Most of us still have good friends who have been in our lives for a long time. These

friends don't question us when we drink water at the dinner table. They care about our welfare at least as much as we do ourselves and accept our new way of life as correct for us.

Ever since we left school, we had always met up on a Friday night to get drunk, have a dance and a laugh. I came to AA and could see that I had a drink problem, but the people seemed so old that I couldn't imagine spending all of my evenings with them. Once I felt strong enough, I turned up on a Friday to surprise my friends and show them how much I had changed. We had a laugh and I found that I didn't need to drink to get on the dance floor. I enjoyed it so much that Friday night started to become a part of my life again. I felt that because I was sober I might also be a good influence on a couple in the gang who were starting to have problems. I got one of them to come to a meeting and I tried to talk about AA, but they laughed at me and so I never mentioned it to them again. I knew that the people at AA would not understand that I felt I was doing some good as well as enjoying myself, so I didn't talk about Friday night with them. I felt confident that I could keep both sides of my life separate without it becoming a problem.

It went wrong late one Friday, in a club, chatting to a couple of lads. My friend, who was drunk, pushed in and said "Don't talk to her, she's a nun, doesn't drink, says her prayers, you need somebody who is up for a laugh". I was hurt and furious and started downing drinks like there was no tomorrow, in fact there wasn't. Tomorrow or the next day did not exist until I came around in the hospital three days later. Hindsight is often extremely clear. The fact that I decided to keep my Friday nights secret should have set off alarm bells, in fact, it had, but I didn't want to lose my fun night out.

Obsessions: Alcoholics seem to be able to develop obsessions for just about anything. It could be buying a new pair of shoes or a bread-making machine. Once we have made a decision that we need something, we have to have it and have it now! For simple things like shoes or bread making this is not usually a problem, we can laugh about how we sat up all night searching the Internet in our quest for the perfect answer. However, this can slip over into more disturbing behaviour when directed at other things.

An obsession for another person can prove quite frightening for both the object and the onlookers, but we tend not to see what we are doing. To us we are merely exhibiting love and affection. The "buzz" of infatuation is addictive and when we feel thwarted in our current obsession, life becomes flat. We look around for something to re-ignite the spark and the ever-present whispers can take us in the direction of a drink. Possibly, not in a direct way, but thoughts along the lines of "I'll show them" will start us on the track towards misery again.

Inventory taking: It is difficult to avoid falling into the trap of taking other peoples inventories. This curse plagues us from joining the fellowship through to the grave. We can justify it, claiming that we are examining their behaviour so that we can be more helpful to them, but we are usually either gloating over their misfortune, or gossiping (in a well-meaning way…) about them. It is too easy to sit in judgement of somebody without asking the question, "What experience took the blank page of a young child and created somebody who reacts this way?" We rarely know the details of a person's past (or present), but does this prevent our judgement? Engrossed in the inventory of others, we completely disregard our own shortcomings.

…And when we were wrong promptly admitted it.

The monkey is waiting patiently to trap us into wrong behaviour. This is why it is so important to keep talking to other recovering alcoholics openly and honestly about what we are doing. By dropping our mask and exposing our current desires and objectives, we allow others to see what we cannot see for ourselves. If we become unable to share at a meeting, the illness has succeeded in driving a wedge between recovery and us. If we have done something wrong there are usually four places where we need to admit it; to ourselves, our Higher Power, our AA meeting and to the person that we have wronged. Possibly, all that is required is an apology, or we may realise that our actions have drifted a long way from the principles we are trying to live by. We come to accept that this maintenance is a part of our life and value the ability to review and change our behaviour. When we resent change, it can be a sign that a serious defect is returning.

Review summary (The Promises)

In the first chapter, we introduced a section of the AA book referred to as the promises, when we first looked at them perhaps they seemed an impossible set of dreams.

> We are going to know a new freedom and a new happiness. We will not regret the past nor wish to shut the door on it. We will comprehend the word serenity and we will know peace. No matter how far down the scale we have gone, we will see how our experience can benefit others. That feeling of uselessness and self-pity will disappear. We will lose interest in selfish things and gain interest in our fellows. Self-seeking will slip away. Our whole attitude and outlook upon life will change. Fear of people and economic insecurity will leave us. We will intuitively know how to handle situations which used to baffle us.

(Big Book Alcoholics Anonymous)

By continuing to place our recovery first, we allow our sobriety, spirituality and serenity to grow. There is no great secret or mystery, *don't drink and don't die* is how we become AA old-timers.

Step Eleven

Finding time for Serenity

As practising alcoholics, we rarely stopped to consider anything. As part of our maintenance plan, we need to put in place a quiet time to reflect upon our behaviour. We are now successfully handling all that life throws at us. Unfortunately, we can drift and revert to handling things in our old manner. It would be foolish to think that our ingrained behaviour has gone and will never again resurface. It is through the practise of step eleven that we keep our destructive instincts under control.

Sought through prayer and meditation to improve our conscious contact with God, as we understood Him, praying only for knowledge of His will for us and the power to carry that out.

This step is near the end of the program not at the beginning. Before working through the earlier steps, the monkey can trip us up with words like prayer, meditation and Higher Power in two ways. We might have already tried a spiritual solution to our life problems and we can become convinced that this is the "real" program and ignore the rest. Alternatively, we can refuse to consider prayer and meditation and feel challenged by the suggestion of adopting such superstitious nonsense. Regardless of at which end of the spectrum we find ourselves, step eleven is part of the program. It isn't all of it, but it certainly isn't an optional extra.

Sought through prayer and meditation...

Although the words prayer and meditation seem joined, they aren't, they are two separate concepts. Whilst many people do allow themselves sufficient time to practise both elements together, others find this difficult. We can choose to pray at one point in the day and to meditate at another. It is irrelevant which part of the day we use for which activity – *it is doing it that counts!* Although we can alter how we do this as our needs and abilities change, we should try to find a routine. Planning to "squeeze in" communicating with our higher power when we get a few spare minutes rarely works and demonstrates a lack of humility.

Prayer is simply forming our queries and fears into a logical statement that can be verbalised. Some who reach step eleven adopt a "spiritual" higher power and use prayer as a means of communication. If we are using the group as our Higher Power, we can use prayer as a way of organising our thoughts regarding issues we are anxious about. Many chose to pray at the end of the day asking for help with any issues they feel are causing a problem. Possibly, a specific defect is reoccurring, such as becoming angry or resentful at the way other people seem to be treating us. During our prayer, we can ask for guidance about handling the problem.

Meditation has two phases, a calming phase where we quiet our mind and a focused phase where we use this calmed state to work on a specific problem. Mention meditation to people who have no concept of it and they will immediately react by commenting about crossed legs and saying "Ommm". Whilst all spiritual teachings and many psychological therapies recognise the value of meditation, we immediately belittle it based upon knowledge gleaned from hearsay, television and films. If the monkey can lead us into mocking the idea before we understand it, we remain lost and unable to complete the program.

Meditating as we start the day can make it more organised. Our old way was possibly to launch into the first job that we encountered and rush through the day skipping from task to task like a bumblebee amongst summer flowers. We fall into bed feeling that we have worked as hard as we possibly can, but we often realise we missed something important. We could pass this off as part of leading a busy life, or we can consider changing.

...to improve our conscious contact with God (As we understood Him)

This statement is extremely clear. We are looking to improve and not simply repeat the same old prayer each day. We often realise that the monkey has tricked us. We thought that we were practising our eleventh step because believed we were spending time in prayer. We discover what we had actually been doing was reciting words, echoing little more than a grown up version of, "God bless Mummy, God bless Daddy and can I have a puppy". Having presented our shopping list of demands and wishes, we then get on with life feeling that we have done our "duty".

A closed mind allows our old opinions to reclaim their domination of our outlook. At the start of the program, we have the advantage of our rock bottom to open our mind to new ideas, but towards the end of working through the program, we can close it again in the belief that we have walked the path and that our path is correct. We improve by making effort and by challenging ourselves to move forwards, in doing so we become more open to growth. We could try to read something inspirational, or consciously examine why somebody or something is causing us to feel uneasy. Remember that within the framework of the program our most reliable contact with our Higher Power is through contact with others. We could take time to talk to people with a different set of beliefs and try to understand their point of view. If we undertake this with a spirit of humility, charity and compassion, we often find life becomes more satisfying and less motivated by self.

How much time are we willing to commit to prayer and meditation?

When we consider this question, most of us discover that we begrudge allowing time measured in minutes. This is strange when we assess how much time we squandered drinking. Not counting the amount of time taken to acquire drink and to be sociable, we could try to estimate how much time we spent with alcohol actually in our hand. It seems reasonable to ask that we dedicate at least this amount of time each day towards our recovery. Even though alcoholics are supposed to be selfish and self-centred, we often find it difficult to take some time for ourselves. We feel that we are so busy in our daily life that we cannot consider wasting time sitting and doing nothing. *Step Eleven is not simply sitting and thinking. It is making a commitment to dedicate part of our day to self-care.*

It can be a dangerous way of thinking to use the excuse that we are having some quiet time for ourselves rather than going to a meeting. We need to be willing to change the balance of our day so that we can fit all aspects of our recovery into it in a planned and unhurried manner. We have our priorities wrong if we are not capable of allowing time for meetings, work, our family and us.

If we take the time to pray and meditate and life improves, how do we react? As alcoholics, we can have a tendency towards thinking that if something makes us feel good then by doubling the dose we will feel even better. Sadly, we don't apply this to a positive activity such as prayer and meditation. Once we are feeling good, the monkey starts to distract us by filling our lives and we are tempted into reducing the amount of time spent practising our eleventh step, or even start to skip it entirely.

...praying only for knowledge of His will for us...

Although the word prayer can seem frightening, it still works on a completely secular level. If our Higher Power is the meeting, what is the meeting's will for us? The meeting wants us to get well. It wants us to be able to live our life in a comfortable and pleasant manner. The meeting certainly wants us to evolve into becoming one of the people "with a sobriety you can admire". It is only by people continuing to grow into sobriety that the meeting survives.

In addition to aspirations for our development, the meeting has its own changing needs regarding our role. As we progress, it might need us to become more actively involved in helping it to run. As time passes, we need to relinquish office and allow others to move into such positions so that they can grow.

Secular or spiritual, the important statement is that we seek only "knowledge of His will for us". It is too easy for anything else to become "our will for him". We don't always know what Gods will is for us, but our conscience is usually able to tell us what it isn't.

...and the power to carry that out.

There are times when we are frightened about how life seems to be unfolding and we start to doubt the value of continuing. It is at these times we need the confidence that we will reach the end of the tunnel and it will then be obvious why it was necessary. If we are certain we are acting in good faith, then we can be confident that we will have the strength to see through whatever is necessary.

A meditation to start the day

The idea that meditation can have two phases comes as a surprise to many people. We all know about the relaxing phase, but rarely learn techniques to use this mental state to focus. Below is an example of a meditation exercise, but if this doesn't work, don't give up too quickly. There are lessons, books and audio's available to help. Don't be scared to talk to others, very few of us arrive with a full knowledge of how to meditate. Even when we believe we do, it is a good idea to check what we are doing and make sure that we are not tricking ourselves into thinking we can have an easy ride in this part of the program.

Sit upright, but relaxed, we don't want to risk dozing off. If we concentrate on breathing slowly and deeper than normal, we relax; breathing and learning to examine our body mentally for areas of tension are essential skills to master.

Close your eyes and cast your mind out. Try to catch the sounds from far away, listen to the rumble of the trucks, the strange noises usually present. Be aware of them, not focused upon them. After two-three minutes, move your hearing into the room, listen to the noises, a clock ticking, the plaster cracking, note them but do not focus, hold this awareness again for two-three minutes, at all times keep your breathing regular, deep and steady. Finally move your hearing into your head. Listen to the noises, notice the hiss of blood in your ears, be aware, not focused. Move the focus of your senses forwards into your nose, feel the air as it runs against the skin of your nostrils and breathe steadily.

Imagine a cloud floating in front of you. It is a pleasant and relaxing colour. Inhale this cloud, imagining that it swirls into your head displacing "blackness". As you exhale, "see" the

blackness drift away, leaving your head filled with the colour.
Repeat the exercise five times and then do the same to each part
of your body, neck, shoulders, arms, chest, stomach etc. Each
time fill with the colour, exhale the tension, and relax as you
breathe out a black cloud.

At this point, thoughts will start to push into your
consciousness. When you recognise them, let them go, do not
pursue them, enjoy the peace of not having any "real" thoughts
going on. After a time, gradually bring yourself back into
allowing the plan of the day to come into focus. What are you
going to do? What situations require decisions? Which of these
decisions are you equipped to make, which require further
investigation? What sort of investigation should you
undertake? Should you pass certain problems to others? Are
the problems yours to carry in the first place? Should you hand
them over to your Higher Power to handle? Edge your thinking
back up into full consciousness and feel ready to face the day.

Daily Growth

The objective of this step is to allow us to grow as people.
As practicing alcoholics, we tend to have stunted our
emotional growth, like plants growing in soil too shallow,
we were unable to take root and reach our full potential.
We have now been replanted into a more fertile and
suitable location. Any gardener will tell you that it takes
time for such a plant to recover, but given time and help, a
plant can grow back to a full and healthy state.

As our sobriety unfolds, we start to see that it has been our
own expectations that have held us back. We can start to
grow beyond anything we thought possible. Rather like if
we had spent our life living in a tent, we would be able to
imagine a bigger tent, but we could never conceive a
mansion made of brick. The same is true for our
perception of a way of life. By developing the humility to
accept external guidance and influence, we allow

ourselves to grow into a way of life – Beyond our wildest dreams.

Summary Questions:

- Have I chosen a time of day to pray and meditate?

- How many times in the last seven days did I achieve this?

- Can I improve what I am doing?

- Have I changed any part of my life based upon my prayer and meditation?

Step Twelve

So that's it then?

The house is built, the course is run, and all of the other mixed metaphors are completed. It is at the twelfth step that we pull all of the elements of the program together and complete our framework for life.

Having had a spiritual awakening as the result of these steps, we tried to carry this message to alcoholics, and to practice these principles in all our affairs.

We often use "Twelfth Step" as short hand for working with others and we hear visiting somebody who has called the help line described as going on a "twelfth step call". In reality, the twelfth step is much bigger; it suggests how we should continue to live our lives. We can break it down into individual phrases and check that we are comfortable with them.

Having had a spiritual awakening...

The term spiritual awakening means that we now base our life upon spiritual principles. The foundations of these principles are humility, honesty and compassion. We are not the centre of the universe and we accept that others have as much right to be here. We recognise that we don't have to be self-sufficient in all things and that we can reply upon an outside power. This power will provide support and guidance in our life, *to any extent we will allow*.

Snakes and Ladders

If spiritual concepts are still causing any discomfort, we are probably not ready to work through step twelve and should try backtracking over the steps to find out where we missed the path. How could we have thoroughly done step nine and achieved a fundamental change without accepting spiritual principles? How could we have humbly asked to remove our defects in step seven? How could we have made a decision to turn our will and our life over, in step three? How could we have come to believe that a power greater than ourselves could restore us to sanity, in step two?

The monkey plays games with us and we can think of this as Snakes and Ladders. Just as we thought we had climbed the ladder of the twelve steps, we hit a snake that slides us all the way back to the start. Although it is essential that we complete the program in sequence, we now see that the program is not a "grading system". Maths lessons start by teaching us how to add simple numbers together. We then progress to subtraction, multiplication and division. It would seem degrading if we were sent back to learn how to add up again after reaching the stage of advanced calculus.

This is not the case with the program. Whilst step one should always be practised with "hundred percent acceptance" *we admitted we were powerless over alcohol – that our lives had become unmanageable*, it is common to realise that our willingness to hand over our lives has slipped away or that we have hurt other people and have not made amends for doing so. It is a life long program. Step eight is no more important or complex than step three. All of the steps have their place in our daily life and we constantly call upon the lessons embodied within each of them.

...as the result of these steps...

We often ended up at the doors of AA because we thought

we were "Special" and "Different" and even at the end of the program, we can become diverted by this style of thinking. This step states that we have our spiritual awakening as *the* result of following the program. A few of us experience a thunderous and inspirational awakening, but we are falling for a trick of the monkey when we hope for something that removes the need to work diligently through all of the steps.

...We tried to carry this message to alcoholics...

The step quite specifically does not say, help, save or rescue. The only message we have is that the program of AA worked for us. The people we visit are free to continue to drink and die. It is not our role to get them sober. It is essential to remember that step twelve exists in the program that we are doing - it is our step twelve.

It is common to hear people say that they are not being successful at carrying the message and that people they talk to fail to stop drinking. This will frequently be the case, but we simply try to carry the message. We might want to do other things, but that is not part of the twelfth step. Many arrive at the door of the fellowship wanting somebody else to take responsibility for their illness. They want a magic pill or a ritual that will fix them when everything else has failed. It is essential to allow people to stand on their own two feet. We show them that it worked for us and they can choose to recover if they want to.

Being there for the newcomer

Most of us are apprehensive when we go to our initial meeting. Ideally, the first contact a newcomer should have with AA is a sober person holding out their hand in friendship. We go to meetings for ourselves, but we have a responsibility to provide the newcomer with their best possible chance to recover.

If the person from AA attending a "Twelfth step call" appears to be eccentric in their appearance or behaviour, they can be off-putting. Whilst we feel we are being ourselves wearing worn out jeans and a leather motorcycle jacket, we must be conscious of the impression we are projecting to the person in front of us. We don't need to turn up looking like tailors dummies, but some thought about our outward appearance goes a long way towards calming a nervous newcomer.

If we experienced the handshake offered by strangers and the comforting nods as we poured out our heart, then we should provide this without question. We have received a precious gift in sobriety and the best way we know to keep this gift is to be willing to give it away to other people.

What can I say?

A person who has no knowledge of AA or of the illness of alcoholism can be antagonistic towards somebody who appears to be a do-gooder with a lecture. The chances are that family and friends have repeatedly told them to "pull themselves together". Their last chance seems to be reaching out to AA.

When we visit somebody in their home, it is important to encourage them to talk. Once they start, we can then expose elements of our own story that they can identify with. The strange fact is that a sober alcoholic can establish a rapport with a suffering one incredibly quickly.

All that is required is a simple display of the principles that saved our lives and the offer that they can follow the same path. If the person wants to argue and debate, we can point out that we used to do that, but no longer do so.

It is pointless trying to argue somebody into sobriety and it will be damaging in the end.

Sometimes we feel that we have something important to share for the newcomer at a meeting. We must be careful about hogging the time in an attempt to make our point. We really don't know what it is the newcomer needs to hear to save their life and it is better to allow a meeting to proceed naturally. Although there is little difference between the male or female shares, we don't know this at our first meeting. When possible, we should allow them to hear some same sex shares either by sharing or remaining quiet, even when we don't want to.

We must always remember that we are dealing with people's lives. We have the power to kill by our unguarded statements. Our opinions are dangerous and we should almost certainly not discuss them with somebody when we are attending a twelfth step call. If we stick to the time-honoured script of Experience, Strength and Hope and nothing else, we can be confident that we are offering them their best possible chance of recovery.

When can I start doing this on my own?

It is unwise to attend a twelfth step on our own, regardless of length of time in the fellowship. There are times when this will happen, but it should not be normal behaviour, certainly never with the opposite sex. This is to protect both parties and the reputation of AA. A person making their first call for help can be in an unpredictably fragile state and we may encounter something outside of our control and experience.

Keep going to meetings.

Regardless of how long we have been around, it is part of

our twelfth step to keep going to meetings. One of the greatest tricks of the monkey is to let us work through the program and then to attract us away. We fill our lives with important and interesting activities and we start to feel that we cannot spare the time to attend meetings. We justify this by claiming that we came to the meetings to enable us to rejoin normal life. *This is not true.* We came to stop drinking and it is important that we continue to turn up not just for our own well-being, but to give back something given freely to us. As a responsible member, we should try to:

Turn up on time so that the meeting can commence promptly without disruption. Nobody can avoid being late occasionally, but if we realise that we are always the last person into the room we need to question and change our behaviour.

Share openly to make sure we keep ourselves in perspective and to allow other people to identify with our story. We don't know what element of our journey will be the meaningful trigger that somebody identifies with.

Be approachable. We can become engrossed in "catching up" with friends at the meeting and assume that somebody else will talk to the newcomer. It is intimidating for them to break into a conversation and easy for them to feel rejected.

By being there and available we provide the gift of support and this should never be underestimated.

...And to practice these principles in all our affairs.

It is easy to use the words "living in the program", but what is really meant by this statement? By practicing the opposite of our known defects and adopting the activities of steps ten, eleven and twelve we make sure we remain a fully functioning worthwhile member of society. As time passes, the positive aspects of our personality will show through and people will begin to see us as a "sober" person.

Humility: Without humility, people will not see much of a change in our behaviour. We should have ceased to offer uneducated opinions to those around us, but be willing to shoulder responsibility as required. We should always keep an eye on our motives. If we are successful, others come to rely on our sober judgement and action in a way that we would not have thought possible. We can be part of a team without needing to be the star and take real satisfaction on the day that they credit another member of the team with something we did and we don't immediately demand the recognition.

Honesty: Self-honesty, visible to everybody we meet is a habit that will become second nature to us. We leave our fantasy world behind and fit in to reality.

Moderation: Life is more peaceful when we are content with what we need, rather than desperate for what we want. By replacing our greed with moderate behaviour, we see that our needs are usually within our reach whereas our "wants" rarely are.

Self-Awareness: Only by considering our own needs as much as we consider the needs of our family and friends can we continue to grow and successfully practice the twelfth step. We don't have infinite resources and if we drain them, old thinking rushes in to flood our life with chaos.

Compassion: Other people have their right to an opinion

and they can have a bad day without us making it worse
for them. When we are living within the program, it is
difficult to react spitefully to another person. We are able
to hold out our hand to those in trouble and no longer
have a hidden agenda for our behaviour.

Gratitude: When we have it, gratitude for our recovery
would seem fundamental, but it is surprising how often
we forget. We know that we should be grateful for the
new way of life we have, but we can find ourselves
complaining that things are not how we want them to be.

Summary

"Living in the program," means that our actions and
behaviour are those expected of every respectable and
sober member of society. Can we really take pride in
acting normally? Yes, we can. When we started our
recovery, we were living a life so far from these principles
that they were entirely alien concepts. The practice of the
program has transformed us. If we ask how much each of
the words highlighted above was a part of the "old us" we
can see how much we have changed.

It will take time for those close to us to gain the confidence
that we are serious about our new behaviour. They are the
people who bore the brunt of our actions in the past and
will be the last to acknowledge the change. It can take
years of consistently demonstrating our recovery before
they are convinced, but we shouldn't be discouraged.
Although we desperately want these people to accept us
as we now are, we will merely harden their attitude
against us if we try to demand that they do so.

In time, people recognise that the drunken liability of old
has now become a worthwhile person. They don't know
how this change has occurred, but they can see that it is

the case. We start out on the journey through the steps because we have to. When we reach the end of the steps, we continue with them because we want to. There will be times when we have problems and we always have a choice about how we will face them:

- We can face them with a clear and sober mind with the strength of other recovering alcoholics and a Higher Power to lean on.

- We can face them alone, drunk and befuddled with a monkey swinging from our neck screaming insane directions at us.

Remember that this choice presented a dilemma when we started the journey.

Final questions...

- Have I resisted being dishonest for self-gain today?

- Have I held out my hand to somebody today?

- Have I avoided mocking or judging other people today?

- Have I been grateful for my life today?

If the answer to these has been yes, then today should have been a good day.

Pulling it together

Cookery is a good analogy for how we learn to live a sober life, not the precise art of bread making, but the more flexible dishes such as stew, curry or chow mein. With these dishes, we can adjust the basic ingredients as we go along to end up with an acceptable dish. The same is true of living a sober life. Provided we have the basic ingredients, we can adjust the quantities as we go.

If all that was required was an understanding of the program of AA we could recover by simply reading it in the comfort of our own home, but the basic ingredients of a sober life are the program, meetings and people. In the first part of the book, we discussed the program. In this next section, we will discuss meetings and people.

Meetings

A person would have to have lived a cut off existence never to have seen a representation of AA in film or on television. We often have preconceptions of what occurs at an AA meeting and virtually all of them are wrong. We picture a room full of slightly down at heel eccentric characters all waiting for the opportunity to speak whilst being lectured from the front of the room. Secretly, we might hope that amongst these oddball characters we will find the hidden gem of a person who will offer the romantic relationship that has so far eluded us.

When we attend our first AA meetings, we come across people who proclaim that they have not had a drink for over twenty years and yet attend meetings every week. We probably anticipated attending once a week for a few months and then we would be free to get on with our life. We may well hope to arrange for "private sessions" rather than attending a public group, but they tell us that this is not how AA works. It is vitally important that we deflate our ego and quickly change from thinking how special we are into accepting that we are "just another drunk" in the room.

The analogy of the dialysis machine explains a good attitude towards going to meetings:

Somebody who needs dialysis accepts regular connection to a machine. They can argue if they like and refuse to go, but they will die a horrible and unnecessary death. An AA meeting is not as traumatic as dialysis, it doesn't require surgery to "plumb" in the fittings, but without meetings, we risk dying a horrible and unnecessary death.

The illness often convinces us that this is being overdramatic and that we are not risking death at all. We cite the example of old "Uncle Albert" who drank a bottle of whisky every day until his death at the age of ninety-nine and convince ourselves that we are from "strong stock" and perfectly capable of carrying on the family tradition.

I had tried and given up on AA many years before I stopped drinking for the final time. This time I had been hospitalised and upon release, told to get back to AA. I rebelled for a short period, but I knew that I was getting close to drinking again, this would be the final straw for my family and so I went. After the meeting, somebody told me to get to ninety meetings in ninety days if I wanted to get sober. My answer was "Oh, now I am sober my wife likes to have me around the house and she would be upset if I went out so frequently."

I have no idea where this came from, my wife despised me and my daughters had disowned me, my time was my own to do what I liked with. Strangely, the next day I did go to another meeting, then another and another. I didn't achieve ninety in ninety, but I did make over seventy. A few years on, I still attend five a week, not because I have to, but because I want to.

It took a long time for my family to start to accept me again, but it happened. At the christening of my first grandchild, I cried with happiness at what the guidance of the meetings had given to me, not just freedom from drinking, but a completely new chance at life.

Why people feel unable to go to meetings.

At first, the idea of going to meetings on a regular basis seems ridiculous and these are some of the common objections raised when people are justifying why they cannot go to meetings:

Too busy, "I'm too busy to go to meetings," springs into our mind. Some of us are working hard to prove how valuable we are, others just feel pressure from our daily chaos. For many of us there is just not enough time in the day and the idea of sacrificing more of it by going to meetings seems too much to ask.

We solve the claim of being too busy by continuing to drink after the point that we should stop. Alcohol makes an ideal cleaning fluid and eventually we use it to scrub away the important job, family, friends and social activities. The absurdity of this excuse is that we rarely appreciate how close to death we really are. If we did, we would see that the things making us busy aren't worth sacrificing our lives over.

Pride, "I don't want strangers knowing about my life", although we frequently unfold our tale of woe to the stranger on the next bar stool, it seems too degrading to formalise this process. This statement shows just how important we feel we are. Do we truly believe that strangers are waiting to hear our story so that they can besmirch our good name? Thoughts like, "people with nothing better to do than sit around gossiping…" sometimes occur, but secretly, we are probably clinging to the hope that we will repair the damage and cover it up before anybody knows about it.

Shame, occurs when we feel people can see what we don't like about ourselves. Our defensive shell is penetrated and finding ourselves unexpectedly exposed we become self-conscious. We think that we have been clever in concealing the depths of our problems, but do we genuinely believe that nobody knows that we have a drink problem? Family, friends, work colleagues and strangers are all painfully aware of our plight. In fact, we are usually the last person to acknowledge it.

Self-Deception, "My problems are different from theirs so they won't be able to help me." We feel that we are the only ones facing our specific problems such as, lost jobs, lost wives and lost families. Alone, our lives seem destroyed and thinking that we drink for different reasons than anybody else, we convince ourselves to remain isolated in the darkness of our imagined uniqueness.

Fear, we can be scared of attending meetings in our own area because we don't want people to see us. Thankfully, there are so many venues that we don't have to go to the one closest to home if we don't want to. Our fears may prove foolish, but it is better to travel, than not to go at all. There can be some justification if we have to deal with alcoholics on a professional basis. A counsellor or a doctor doesn't want to feel the need to put on a "brave face" if they encounter their own patients, but for the rest of us, our fears subside and drop away. The pleasure of being able to walk, rather than drive to a meeting normally outweighs any fear of criticism. After all, did making a fool of ourselves stop us before? Fighting, causing a scene, or covering ourselves in vomit, didn't keep us away for long. Why then would we be scared to be seen getting help to sort out our lives? Possibly, we want to make sure that we have a way back into our old life should we decide that AA isn't right for us.

Why we should go to meetings

The important action is to identify some meetings that we can attend. "Ninety meetings in ninety days, if you don't like what you see then we refund your misery," is an often-heard saying. It is important to make the commitment to get to meetings and try to become part of the "fellowship" of AA.

Our attitude needs to stay fresh for the rest of our lives and there is a regular pattern seen at most meetings. Look at the people who stay behind to talk after the formal part of the meeting. If we go back to the meeting five years later, we will see the same faces doing the same thing. There will have been a hundred faces come and gone during the five years, but these people survived, proving that those who are actively involved with others stay sober.

There are many reasons why we should attend meetings and here are a few.

Humility, not to be confused with Humiliation, the emotion we feel if we expose ourselves to ridicule. A meeting never judges us, we share to we keep ourselves in perspective, gaining insight into a "modest sense of our own true worth".

Guidance, through exposing our shortcomings and feelings we make it possible for other people to help and guide us. How could they know that we are heading down a dangerous path if we don't tell them what we are planning? Somebody in the room will have tried whatever seems a bright idea to us and they will be able to point out the pitfall in our plans.

Gratitude, towards the people who freely gave their own time to our recovery, it is often said that it is impossible to drink when we are grateful for our sobriety.

Support, even if we don't feel we have anything to offer, by stopping drinking and attending our second and subsequent meetings, we give hope to others. It can be overwhelming for a newcomer to conceive of twenty years without a drink, but they get hope when they see somebody who has achieved a week. Similarly, somebody with five years gives hope to people with two years, the ten year old to the five year old and so on.

Companionship, we soon realise that drunks are boring to sober people and whilst we all have friends outside the fellowship of AA, these are not the "fair weather" friends from the pub. The people at the meetings soon become closer than we could imagine and we understand what friendship is really about.

Commitment, we stay safe when we continue to remind ourselves about the seriousness of our illness. There can be no argument or discussion about attending meetings. We need to get to as many as we can sensibly attend because without remaining fully committed to recovery, we will fail. This is especially true when we start to justify why it makes sense not to go. "It's too cold / late", "I'm too tired" are possibly signs of a problem.

Why do people stop going to meetings?

There isn't a definitive answer to this, but a common

theme is a tendency to allow living to become more important than *sober living*.

Life got too comfortable, if sitting in the meeting and not sharing becomes too comfortable, the monkey will convince us that we are not gaining anything from being there. We cut down on our meetings, but tell ourselves that we are still following the program and continue the justification even when we finally tail off to not attending any at all.

Complacency, life had once seemed finished, but as our minds clear and things improve, we seem to run out of time. We decide that we can cut down on going to meetings and talking with sober alcoholics. We reason that now we are sober we want to live our lives to the full.

Our problem is that our vision of "living life to the full" can be unrealistic and involve activities any sober person wouldn't consider. We start to believe that we can run on the edge and freely mix with drinking people. If anybody challenges us, we tell them "I didn't get sober to hide away in meetings", brushing aside any concerns they harbour. As we do so, things that had been unacceptable creep back in to become acceptable. Each line we cross adds another barrier between sobriety and us.

Secrets mean that we don't want to share in the meeting because "they will not understand". By not being able to share openly, we continually share the same old stories from our past, failing to reveal what is really happening in our lives. Because we get nothing from sharing, the meeting seems to drag and we decide to cut down on them claiming that they don't work any more.

Pride often gets in the way of honest sharing. We sometimes feel that the meeting is unfairly judging us and rather than accept the criticism we either clam up or stop attending.

Are the meetings perfect?

It would be great to say that AA and the meetings exist untainted without a hint of ego and politics, but meetings involve people and people get things wrong. Common examples are dominating the meeting with overtly religious attitudes or trying to form specialist groups, such as "young, single, left handed, tall people" meetings. Most of what is proposed sounds attractive and plausible. After all, what is wrong with wanting a meeting made up of "like-minded" people?

Problems occur when we want to exclude people from "our" meeting. All too easily, intolerance draws us into judging people as not "the right sort". The basis of the judgement can be skin colour or religion. It can be their social background or colourful vocabulary. It can be as simple as wanting single sex meetings. It is ridiculous, but more than one meeting has suggested refusing entrance to people who have been drinking that day.

Soon after the start of AA, they found they needed guidelines to help people keep the meetings free from restrictive and damaging behaviour. The "Traditions" of AA embody these guidelines and maintaining them is as important to our common welfare as the program is to our individual recovery. We should avoid meetings that stray from the Traditions of AA. Over time, either they will correct themselves, or because people stop attending them, they fail and close.

The Twelve Traditions

1.   Our common welfare should come first; personal

recovery depends upon A.A. unity.

2.   For our group purpose, there is but one ultimate authority, a loving God as He may express Himself in our group conscience. Our leaders are but trusted servants; they do not govern.

3.   The only requirement for A.A. membership is a desire to stop drinking.

4.   Each group should be autonomous except in matters affecting other groups or A.A. as a whole.

5.   Each group has but one primary purpose, to carry its message to the alcoholic who still suffers.

6.   An A.A. group ought never endorse, finance, or lend the A.A. name to any related facility or outside enterprise, lest problems of money, property, and prestige divert us from our primary purpose.

7.   Every A.A. group ought to be fully self-supporting, declining outside contributions.

8.   Alcoholics Anonymous should remain forever non-professional, but our service centres may employ special workers.

9.   A.A., as such, ought never be organized, but we may create service boards or committees directly responsible to those they serve.

10.   Alcoholics Anonymous has no opinion on outside issues; hence the A.A. name ought never be drawn into public controversy.

11.   Our public relations policy is based on attraction rather than promotion; we need always maintain

personal anonymity at the level of press, radio, and films.

12.   Anonymity is the spiritual foundation of all our traditions, ever reminding us to place principles before personalities.

Finding a home group

A meeting should have the same personality we look for in a close friend or sponsor within AA. It should be approachable and able to guide us when we stray from the program. We should be able to share and feel safe that what we say in the meeting will stay in the meeting.

When we find a group that feels like a sponsor, we should consider making it our home group. A home group is simply a meeting we make a commitment to attending. This group of people will watch us mature from our shaky start into a fully committed member of AA. These strangers often know more about us than our own family do and they can challenge us when they see that we are not functioning within the principles of the program. A home group is a guardian to watch over us and help us to stay on course. We all waver at times and this is frequently apparent to others a long time before we know about it.

People

The people at a meeting usually come from a broader background than encountered under any other circumstances. The illness is the same whether we drink rough alcohol or champagne and the characters at the meeting range from thieves to priests, tramps to millionaires. These unlikely companions make up the

Fellowship of AA. Regardless of their background, there are two absolute truths:

- We are all Alcoholics

- We are all at some stage of recovery or relapse.

To put it another way, there are no bosses or professionals to tell us what we "should" be doing and because we all suffer from the illness of alcoholism, we all need help and support to remain well.

There will be people we find physically or emotionally attractive and others who seem downright scary. We will listen to some who bore or revolt us and encounter many who enthral and entertain. At first, we think that we will have more in common with people who have only been sober for a short period. We suspect that those who have been around a long time will not want to be bothered with a newcomer. These thoughts are untrue and dangerous.

It is the monkey tricking us when we decide to strike up a friendship with another newcomer. Other newcomers cannot support us and the meeting is not a social club. We go to meetings to learn how to live a happy sober life and it is far better to talk to somebody who is doing that than to simply find "new pals". People with a long-term sobriety usually enjoy talking with newcomers offering support and experience. We learn to trust that there are people who will put out their hand to somebody without expecting anything in return. Trust does not come easily. Our defects motivated us for so long that we assume everybody else behaves the same way.

People with a sobriety that we admire

It can be puzzling when people tell us not to be

judgemental and to not take other peoples inventories, and then in the next breath tell us to look for *people with a sobriety we admire*. How are we supposed to do this, especially when they tell us that length of time not drinking is no indication of sobriety?

We judge others based upon simple criteria; are they like us? Do they have a nice car or house? Do they have a job we admire? These material criteria don't work well when we are evaluating sobriety, the people who learnt the most during their recovery often fell the farthest.

Few of us arrive readily able to identify spiritual wealth. It takes time to learn how to sit quietly in a room and appreciate the depth of experience other people have to offer. These people may not be the most affluent, or skilled at putting their experience into words, but by ignoring our prejudice, we can see that they do in fact have a better quality of life than ours, even when they don't "measure up" based upon our old standards.

Sharing

We usually envisage other types of meetings as a lot of talking, usually by a few loud voices looking to push through their own agenda. However, at an AA meeting, the focus is upon listening. Even if we have urgent questions or issues, we have to wait our turn and remain silent allowing the current speaker their opportunity to share.

Most of us don't even understand the term "sharing", we think it is the same as talking – and we know how to do that. We often want to dominate, babbling about how badly life has treated us. Somebody may suggest that we "take the cotton wool out of our ears and stuff it in our mouth", although this statement initially hurts us, there are extremely good reasons why this is good advice.

Sharing is in fact a two way process, speaking and listening. The normal person is born with two ears and one mouth and we should use them in these proportions. Whilst it can be therapeutic to talk, we learn by listening. The meeting is a good classroom and we learn about humility and common courtesy. Adopting acceptable behaviour within meetings prepares us to use it in our daily life.

If the monkey can prevent us from learning how to share, it has won the battle, unchanged, we will remain isolated, self-absorbed and sick. When we attend an AA meeting, we are threatening the monkey's habitat and it will play every trick it knows to protect itself. It does this by manipulating our defects to block our ears and keep our mouths closed. The main symptom of these defects is judgement. We judge everyone around us and our judgement holds shut the doorway to growth. If we look deeper into our emotions, the same defects we identified earlier emerge.

Pride surfaces when we want to share and impress the rest of the meeting. We sit planning our share and then afterwards mentally leave the room to think about other things. Possibly, we bask in imagined adoration from the other people in the room who are astounded by our eloquence and depth of knowledge.

Envy dominates us when we judge everybody in the room and decide that because they still have their partners and families that they don't understand the problems that we have to cope with.

Anger rules us when we stop listening because we tell ourselves that that this person or that person has nothing we want to hear or because they seem to be repeating the same old thing time after time.

Identifying what is going on in our own mind is the first step towards correcting this and just as before, the answer is to look for the opposite of the defect. Humility, gratitude, and compassion defuse these negative blocks and allow us to take part in the meeting.

Learning to share is important. To do it we need to be honest with ourselves and effectively give permission to others to be honest with us. We can be embarrassed to try. Overawed by the depth and coherence of what we hear, for the first time in our lives we listen to people speaking honestly about their feelings, pain and fears. We feel that we will never be able to match the honesty and wisdom of these people.

Nobody (except possibly us) expects a performance. We are all drunks trying to stay away from a drink one day at a time. A good starting point is to just join in, announce our name, and confirm that we are alcoholic. Nobody finds it easy and we all have different barriers towards speaking openly in the meeting. If it didn't provide huge rewards, we would not go through with it. Sometimes just sharing the frustrations felt during the day will be sufficient to open the floodgates.

For me to be able to share honestly I have to drop all masks and defences before I start and make a conscious decision to share as me. After saying, "my name is..." I take a short pause and try to confirm that I have locked "The Showman" away. I then have to be open to receiving feedback on whatever I share without being defensive or mentally blocking it because "they don't understand."

Why is anonymity important?

This is one of the questions most people ask when they arrive at the doors of AA, if, as we claim, there is nothing to be embarrassed about in attending the meeting, why the secrecy?

Everybody at the meeting is there for the same reason - to get sober. We all have a sickness and we don't need other prejudices getting in the way of recovery. How easy can it be for a priest to come and talk about not being able to understand the spiritual parts of the program? Who would try to help them understand a Higher Power? Who could talk with a Judge about wisdom or honesty? We all need the freedom to speak openly about our life. Some people will need to talk about degrading experiences and if they fear the consequences, they will not be able to share freely.

We should always respect other people's anonymity. The celebrity who attends a meeting needs as much help and support as any other person. They don't need the stress of their fame getting in the way and they certainly don't need publicity when they go to a meeting. It is tempting to tell people about the famous person we have been sitting with, but somebody we tell, may tell somebody who calls the press. Celebrity or not, what is said in the meeting and who is there should remain there.

Sponsorship

Many people come to meetings, listen and fail because they try to get sober unguided. They usually arrive just as it is starting, bustle to a chair at the back of the room and afterwards they always have somebody waiting or an important event to attend. After a few months, they stop appearing.   We rarely hear from them again, or if we do, we hear that they have left their homes, jobs and families, or died. We never hear that life became so good that they discovered that they didn't need to stop drinking.

Rather than try to invent our own way of recovering, most of us benefit from getting a sponsor. This is simply somebody to guide us through the program and help us to understand the strange feelings and emotions that we experience when we start to live a sober life. When we stop drinking, it is like emerging from a cocoon. Emotions that we didn't know we had start to flicker into existence and "bright" ideas bludgeon into our consciousness. It is rare to meet anybody who has achieved a happy contented sobriety without having a sponsor and it is important to find one.

Finding a sponsor

When we are looking for a sponsor, it is usual to talk with a few people and ask how to do it. One of the confusing clichéd responses to this question is "choose somebody you don't like."   Whilst we are not looking for a new best friend, we are looking for somebody in whom we have confidence.

Occasionally we may encounter somebody who makes us squirm when they share. Each time they open their mouth they seem to be taking our inner most secrets and putting them on the table. This is different from somebody we don't like, this is identifying strongly with another persons experience. A more useful interpretation of the cliché is not that we don't like them, but that they intimidate us. We need to know that they will be willing to hurt our feelings, not because they want to, but because they need to.

Rather than accept a clichéd answer to "how do I find a sponsor," look at the problem a different way. The objective is to learn how to apply the program and live a happy successful life and it is sensible to look for somebody who seems to have achieved this. Sobriety has more depth than not drinking. It means clear thinking and acting responsibly. At first, people who make a lot of noise, but really aren't living by the program can take us in. In the barroom, we claimed to know how to run major corporations and could tell the national football coach exactly how he could win the next major tournament. Alcohol appears to give vast powers of knowledge and skill without us actually needing to learn anything.

We may encounter serial or "professional" sponsors, who appear to sponsor everybody in the area. They may even suggest themselves to us. Whilst there may be nothing wrong in this, is this really what we deserve, to be a battery sponsee?

Although we don't feel it, in the early days of recovery we are vulnerable people. If we were approached by somebody wearing a dirty overcoat and asked "Need a sponsor little (boy / girl)?" it would be easy to spot a potential problem. Unfortunately, such predators do not announce themselves in this way. They seem plausible and concerned for our welfare. Same sex sponsorship is sensible, because it is too easy for the kindness and empathy shown by another person to be confused with something more.

We need somebody we can really talk to, for example, if there is a shared interest in cookery, our sponsor can say something like "working through the program is rather like making a cheese sauce" and illustrate how the raw ingredients, milk, butter, cheese, and flour suddenly combine into a sauce. Whilst this is a great analogy, it is useless if we have never made a cheese sauce.

It is quite normal for sponsorship to evolve into a close and mutually supportive friendship. The "professional" sponsor will not be able to do this, nor will a sponsor we selected because we didn't like them.

To summarise, we are looking for somebody of the same sex, who has done the program, exhibits all the signs of a happy successful life and has the time to talk to us.

It can be surprising when we hear people talk of changing their sponsor. We are not buying a dog - it is not "for life". It is perfectly acceptable to swap sponsors. Sometimes people move away, or we decide that we have more rapport with somebody else. If we approach the change in a sensitive and mature manner, a sponsor will not be hurt or object.

With the help of a sponsor and a few trusted friends, we will be able to establish a routine of attending meetings that will help us develop a happy and enjoyable sobriety.

Recipe for a balanced life

It is now time to put the ingredients together, Program, Meetings, Sponsor and Friends. These soon provide a natural structure and it seems hard to understand how we thought there was a better way to live our lives.

It is impossible to dictate the blend that a specific person needs such as:

- Take one step and work through the detail of it thoroughly each month.

- Add five meetings per week.

- Meet and discuss the program with sponsor in a quiet room once a week.

- Invite two friends per month into our home to allow the detail to settle. (Be willing to reciprocate and visit theirs as well.)

- Once a day take a little time to be quiet and meditate.

It is perfectly acceptable to start with somebody else's recipe and work with that. We soon learn to take these ingredients and create a blend that suits us. Providing that all of the ingredients are included in our life it will work successfully, if it doesn't then we can adjust the quantities a little.

Time to work through the program becomes part of every day. The faster we work through the program and understand it the faster we get better. A step a day is probably too fast, a step a year is probably too slow. Remember that we can decide to do a step again and we have the rest of our life to keep working at it.

Choosing a sponsor, we need to get a sponsor as soon as possible. Remember that if we are tactful and honest it is not a problem to change sponsors later.

Sharing Honestly allows people to see who we really are. It gives people with experience of living sober an insight into how we are living our lives and it gives newcomers hope that they can recover.

People we admire, allow time for people to get to know us, learn to listen and take time to get to know other people. If we allow it to happen, we acquire worthwhile and meaningful friendships with more people than we can possibly imagine.

Number of Meetings, it is easy to reduce the number we attend and difficult to increase it. The best advice is to get to as many meetings as we can sensibly manage. In the early days, this would normally be more than three a week and as we progress rarely less than two a week.

Play the numbers game

If we honestly feel we are living within the guidelines of the program we can have the confidence to say that nobody has the right to tell us to change our lives.

For example, most of us find:

- We need more than one meeting a week.

- It difficult to survive in drinking situations

- As time passes, we need to be more vigilant for the illness creeping back in and poisoning our thoughts.

These are not facts, merely observations. It is true that for every quoted "statistic" we can search around and find the exceptions.

We might meet the lady who has achieved a happy and successful sobriety by attending one meeting a week or the man who enjoys going to nightclubs and dancing until the early hours of the morning. People told them that they were heading for a drink, but they have survived for many years and experience a happy sobriety.

Exceptions always exist, but it is more sensible to accept that we are likely to fail if we fight against the statistics. What kind of guide would let their clients choose a dangerous path without pointing out the safe one other people use?

Training the monkey!

It is impossible to tame a wild animal. The lions at the circus are not tame, but manipulated into performing as though they are. They will maul the lion tamer if he makes a mistake. The circus performer stays safe by keeping their mind on their job when they are in a dangerous situation.

The same is true for the monkey riding on our shoulder. If we stay within sensible boundaries, we are safe. We need to remain aware of our behaviour and make sure that we do not give the monkey an opening through which to attack us. If we get it right, the monkey rides quietly along with us and rarely gets a chance to intrude. To everybody else we appear cured of our incurable illness, but like the lion tamer, pain and death is one slip away.

Rarely have we seen a person fail ...

... who has thoroughly followed our path

The illness lies like a reef beneath the surface of a calm sea.
In good weather, our boat sails cleanly over the hazard,
but in strong tides, the rocks are capable of grinding
mercilessly through the hull of our boat, plunging us into
peril. A good sailor knows where the dangers lie in their
coastal waters and when they must avoid certain stretches.

Chapter five in the Big Book starts with the line: *Rarely
have we seen a person fail who has thoroughly followed our path.*
It is obvious that many people do fail to achieve and
maintain a sober life. Look around the meeting and do
some maths, how many arrive through the doors, how
many stick around? Where do the others go? Sadly, many
give up. Rather than embracing the benefits on offer, they
accept the first glimmerings of a better life and drift away.
It is not just the meetings they abandon, but also the safety
of AA and many find that the illness is waiting for them.

We are never safe

The absolute truth is that regardless of how long we have
been dry, we are never safe from the illness. A fact that
will never change is that the nature of an alcoholic is to
drink. To an outsider it would seem logical that the longer
we remain sober, the easier it gets - this isn't true. An old
timer has to resist all of the temptations that a newcomer
encounters, as well as coping with more subtle ones that
creep in later. Life is like learning a martial art. We learn
moves to counter each ploy our opponent exposes, but a
new trick that we have not encountered before can defeat
us. The monkey can continually bounce us off the mat
whilst we try to discover a counter-move, or we can look

for help. Over time, our knowledge of the game improves, but our opponent, the monkey, is also improving. The final objective of its game is to find a way to make drinking seem acceptable. If we allow this to happen, we are almost certainly heading for a slip – a drink. The term "slip" seems too lightweight for such an enormous event, but seen as an acronym for Sobriety Lost Its Priority, it seems perfect.

Early days

Nobody is motivated into trying AA merely out of a passing interest and we are particularly vulnerable when we first walk through the doors of AA. We are not usually capable of understanding or accepting how serious our illness is and we look for "loop holes" that will allow us to drink again.

Some people arrive apparently determined that they are not going to stop drinking. They might stick around for a short time because they are under the eagle eye of someone who escorts them to meetings, but they listen selectively and use this to justify why AA is wrong for them.

What is there to lose?

Even when we have decided to take it seriously, it can be hard to stay motivated. At the beginning, we can use the number of days we have been sober as a form of incentive. We can tell ourselves that we have achieved "x" days, weeks or months without a drink and we are not willing to waste all of the effort it took to get to this point. The accumulated days in themselves actually count for little. Not drinking one day at a time is essential, but if the only benefit we feel we are getting is that we are not drinking, we will probably start again.

"Just not drinking" is the lowest point we survive at and we all feel this way at times during our recovery. Each day not drinking, we remain clear of insanity, each time we drink, we pull the trigger in our selfish game of Russian roulette. If we can see each day as a contribution towards a better way of life, we are in with a chance.

Failing to accept all of the implications of Alcoholism

A common description of the thinking before embarking on a bout of drinking is the desire to take a holiday from the "AA thing". Although we have stopped drinking, we are usually trying to act the same as we always have. The idea strikes us that just for the one evening we can take a break. We simply want to have our old life back for a short time.

"A" was a man who had achieved great levels of success in his business life and to all of his acquaintances he was a "jolly good chap". If a charity needed somebody to jump out of an airplane or run a marathon to raise funds, "A" was the man. When he returned from each drinking session he proclaimed that it was "too easy" to recover. He explained that if only it would take more than a couple of weeks to recover, he could accept the idea that he was progressively killing himself. At each point in his descent, he failed to attribute the problem to alcoholism. His business failed, but that was the bank and a couple of rogue customers. His jaw was broken in a brawl, but that was simply being in the wrong place at the wrong time. His doctors warned that his heart was failing, but that was merely the "nanny state" trying to restrain a free spirit. Each time he returned he uttered the same plea that he wished it wasn't so easy to recover. Finally, death granted his wish.

"B" was a man who turned things around from living rough on the street. His life improved as he progressed from hostels into dry houses and finally he moved into his own first apartment. He loved where recovery had taken him, but lost control of his finances. After a difficult meeting with his bank manager, he picked up a few cans. They were a way of relieving the tension he was feeling. He didn't want to lose what he had gained, but did not see that they would really harm him that much. He was wrong. He rapidly descended back through the stages he had come up through and ended up back on the street.

Perennial "slippers" attend meetings often proclaiming that they fully understand and appreciate the benefits they are experiencing and then turn up to confess that they have been drinking again.

Whilst these people accept that they have an alcohol problem they don't accept the full implications of step one – *Admitted we were powerless over alcohol and that our lives had become unmanageable*. They admit that they get in a mess when they drink, but assume that they will be able to regain control quickly enough not to do any lasting damage – they are wrong.

Stress and excuses

It is common to believe that drink is the only way to relieve our stress. It sounds acceptable and we can imagine people condoning our actions. Stress is an excuse we have used in the past and this is the most common reason for people to drink on television. We have to accept that we cannot drink – regardless of how we are feeling and that we need to talk to somebody before we do.

A woman felt that she was facing an unsolvable problem. She wanted to install a childproof gate at the bottom of her stairs. Her dilemma was that the fittings would damage the expensive new wallpaper her mother had paid for, but she knew that she wouldn't forgive herself if her child fell down the stairs. The debate seemed to rage inside her head until she screamed for relief.

A woman knew that her husband was out drinking with his friends and felt that it would be stressful when he came home. Her thoughts played and replayed how he would roll in through the door. Each time she went over it the situation got worse until she imagined that they would have a screaming row and that he would beat her senseless. She decided it was better to be drunk when she faced him.

A teacher felt that the government was placing ridiculous demands upon him. At first, he grumbled to his fellow teachers who didn't seem to be willing to take any action. Then he moved on to complaining to his head teacher who listened, but simply replied with the "party line" about how they all had to work under these difficult circumstances. He didn't feel like he could get anybody to take him seriously and finally the frustration seemed to mount out of control and he had to drink.

The ever-present monkey whispers constantly in our ear, "They shouldn't be treating me this way", or "They will criticise me". These are destructive thoughts. We rarely question who "they" are and why they have so much power to unsettle our thinking.

Our need to be right and seen as right can be overpowering. This is simply another incarnation of Pride in our behaviour. Whether we are right or wrong is irrelevant, because we cannot live with conflict for too long. We can remove the danger and disarm these thoughts by letting go and stopping trying to control everything. If we continue to battle with them insisting that we are right then we will almost certainly lose, possibly not just the argument, but our life.

After doing the program

After we have done the program, we are still vulnerable to these early problems, but the excuses can also take on a different form. We are aware that we are alcoholic and that we risk a lot by drinking again. The monkey is always on our shoulder and tricks us into justifying a drink by placing the idea that we can either keep it secret, or that we can return submissively to the meetings having merely lost a little of our time in AA.

It rarely works out this way and if we survive the first occurrence, subsequent ones quickly follow. What had been a "one off" gamble becomes acceptable and we are once again on the merry-go-round of alcoholism. Just like the ride at the fairground, at some point the attendant will appear with their hand outstretched for payment.

Teaching others a lesson/ Cry for help

We can feel that somebody is putting us under too much pressure. This pressure can take many forms. It could be that our partner seems to have dumped a load of household tasks onto us so that we have no time for ourselves. They could have booked to go out with some heavy drinking friends from our past or spent too much money from the joint account. We imagine their mortification when they realise that their behaviour has forced us to throw away our precious sobriety.

Sobriety has a way of making us feel like we can handle any situation life throws at us and we act as though the alcoholic we once were is long gone. In reality, we merely have a thin veneer of sanity, scratch us and the old behaviour is just beneath the surface. We can be suffering, but reluctant to speak out and stand up for our rights. We opt for a more dramatic gesture and justify our action by claiming that we were in so much emotional pain that we had block out the world and our thinking by taking a drink.

A desire to start again

I felt that I had never achieved the levels of happiness that I saw in other people's recovery. Others came in after me and seemed to be able to accept the program without arguing about every tiny detail. They certainly seemed to get a better understanding of higher powers and spirituality than I ever did.

I had been in AA for about six years when I had the bright idea, "Go back drinking and then you can work through the program again and find out where you went wrong". I was quite pleased with this thought, because it seemed so logical and I was sure that my new sponsor would approve because it would give them the chance to guide me through the program from the beginning.

We were driving back from a meeting when I tentatively suggested my good idea. He went quiet and then said, "Why not skip the drinking part? We can pretend that you have already done that and we can start to work through the steps from the beginning". I immediately felt cheated of my justified "last drink" and then I felt a bit stupid for not having come up with the idea myself.

I went through each of the steps again and this time it clicked. I followed the suggestions and stopped arguing about the details. Finally like a light being switched on I grasped the idea of a Higher Power and my sobriety has been a valued gift ever since.

Never abandoning the belief that we "gave up" something

We feel that we are recovering by "running with the hounds", but every so often, our heart desires a jaunt with the foxes. Although we claim to be happy with the way we are now living, we have an underlying belief that we have accepted a second best or crippled existence. When we hear of somebody arranging to do something that we used to enjoy, such as a trip to a sporting event or a night in a jazz club, we suddenly feel left out and envious. These occasions were rarely about the actual event, but about how much alcohol we could consume and although we make a logical decision not to go along, we still feel excluded.

As adolescents, many of us experienced the need to have the right label on our clothes and felt the pressure to show that we were part of the tribe. Now AA awakens our urge to rebel and replaces our parents by forcing us into wearing sensible shoes. Feeling excluded from the "tribe" is a powerful emotion. Not drinking doesn't actually exclude us from much that life offers and contrary to our thinking: *we fit in- until we drink.*

I grew up in one of the toughest parts of the city and I had either to be part of the gang or live in fear. Although I am small, I could fit in because I was bright and I could work things out. I cut the deals for the stolen cars and I held the cash to buy the drugs.

I found myself in AA at an early age and soon I was living a completely different life. I went to college to get an education, but when I looked for jobs, I felt that my background always held me back. I told people how I preferred my life today than where I had been heading, but inside I felt "second class" living on hand-outs.

One night I met the father of one of my old friends and we started to talk. As I walked home, my mind was racing. With all my knowledge, I didn't need to drink or use drugs again and this would make me even sharper. Within a week, I had made some calls and done a couple of break-ins to get some cash. Within two months, I was making money and handling drugs. Within six months I was using and drinking again, I flushed nine years sobriety in less than nine months.

The climb back out of this pit was the hardest thing I ever did. It took me years to recover from the deceit and dishonesty and I can now see how shallow I had been in my original acceptance.

Unwilling to accept defeat

A normal drinker doesn't understand why we would need to "surrender" to drink. For them it is merely a minor part of their entertainment. They may enjoy a nice glass of wine with a meal, or a cool beer whilst relaxing by a sunlit stream. Certainly, it is pleasant, but not worth fighting a battle for.

However, the alcoholic perceives these pleasures as their right and perseveres beyond rational behaviour to maintain them. We imagine ourselves as the battered boxer who refuses to let his corner throw in the towel to save him. In stories, he wins because despite the evidence, he suddenly produces an unexpected recovery to defeat his opponent. Unlike the fantasy of fiction, in real life the battered underdog rarely wins the fight, they simply suffer a deadly beating.

I had always accomplished anything I decided to achieve. I played sport at semi-professional level and I had moved into commerce by turning a failing business into a profit making concern. As a drinker, I prided myself on being able to escort my drunken friends' home at the end of the night.

I started to find myself inexplicably drunk and this led me to talk to my doctor. He explained that I was an alcoholic and suggested I should get treatment. I attended AA, but the idea of stopping completely seemed the attitude of a "quitter". I decided that if I could stop drinking for two years I would prove I could control my drinking. As I approached the end of the two years, I undertook a controlled drinking course that finished shortly before my own deadline. With my usual arrogance, I refused to commence their controlled path until I had completed my target of two years abstinence.

When I tried to control my drinking, I failed. I was convinced there was nothing wrong with the basic plan, it just needed to be refined. I opted for maintaining a cycle of control, decline and clinic. I was in a hotel when I had my last drink. As I raised the glass to my lips, I saw myself reflected in the mirrored wall behind the bar. The man in the mirror looked scared, he knew that he was about to lose control. The humiliation of this final bender stripped all of the excuses away from me. I could not drink and the first one did the damage, regardless of will power, intelligence, planning and money, drink had finally beaten me.

Regardless of how we yearn for the impossible, we have to accept that we cannot do what other people can. People who can't eat seafood don't keep ending up in hospital because they gave it "one last try". If they did, we would consider them insane.

After a long period of sobriety

It seems puzzling that somebody could appear to be a stalwart member of AA and yet end up picking up a drink again. It happens quite frequently, we are all alcoholics and the need to stay away from one drink one day at a time never reduces in importance.

Questionable behaviour

We find ourselves drawn into something that we feel we cannot discuss with our sponsor or friends. It is something that our long experience allows us to justify as acceptable, but we can also see that it could be misinterpreted as dangerous and so we choose to keep quiet. This dishonesty creates a barrier that becomes impossible for us to overcome even when we are regularly attending meetings.

"D" was a woman with eight years sobriety when she discovered alcohol free whisky flavoured drinks. She knew they were safe, but rather than risk any misunderstanding she decided she would keep it a secret. One day she was feeling especially in need of comfort and decided to experiment with a small quantity of the real thing. The experiment went well, nobody noticed and she felt more relaxed than she had done for a long time. With the line crossed, she allowed herself a small drink every day and inevitably lost control.

Her son, who had only been a young child when she came to AA quickly turned upon her. Her husband became cold and dispassionate. He had barely coped with her final drinking days and couldn't go through the lies and deceit again. She was unable to regain sobriety and suffered a miserable existence ended by a fatal fall down a flight of stairs.

"E" had seven years sobriety when she decided it was a good idea to clean out her husband's drinks cabinet and give all of the bottles a polish. Whilst she did this, she decided to take the top off one and sniff the fumes. She didn't drink for a couple of weeks and could justify retrying the experiment with a slight difference. This time she did take a small drink of it, but not enough to affect her. After a couple of months, she had progressed into secret binge drinking. When her family found out, she lost the trust she had built up and subsequently lost everything.

Believing that the program will address any problem

We are encouraged to accept a spiritual awakening, but we can take this to an extreme. We can argue that our Higher Power is capable of anything and can therefore remove our alcoholism completely. Armed with the idea that our Higher Power "watches over us" we can justify any action claiming that if it is not God's will then something will prevent us from proceeding.

After seventeen years, "G" believed that by attending meetings and becoming active in his local church, he achieved not only a reprieve, but attained a full cure from his alcoholism. He started to drink the wine during the blessing with the knowledge that it was the "blood of Christ". He progressed on to accepting a small glass of sherry offered to toast a happy occasion. His drinking quickly ran out of control and the insanity of alcoholism destroyed his home life.

Over his nine-year recovery, "H" had been involved in AA at almost every level of service. His wife felt neglected, met somebody, packed her bags and left. "H" made a great display and proclaimed that the program was there to help him survive anything life threw at him. Even though he attended many meetings, he found himself suffering and isolated, eventually he decided the only option was to drink.

Is there any hope?

Understanding the program is different to practising it. Most of the people in the examples above could quote page numbers from the Big Book, discuss the program and help others to recognise where they were failing.

Practising the program is moving our acceptance out of our heads and into our hearts. Earlier in this book, we saw that all of the world's religions and many practitioners in mental health recognise pride, envy, greed, lust and anger as dangerous traits. The AA program is a way to learn how to adopt their positive opposites into our life. When we accept that vigilance is not a chore, but a necessary part of our life then this statement applies:

"Rarely have we seen a person fail who has thoroughly followed our path"

Staying sober under all conditions

Rabbi Arnold Jacob Wolf explains Jewish spirituality as: walking along a street that's studded with precious stones, and the goal is to gather as many stones as you can or a few of them that are beautiful. The street is three thousand years old, so there are many precious gems in it. Some of the jewels are easily dislodged from the pavement, so you can easily put them into your life, but others will remain stuck in the pavement. Some are so obviously beautiful that you can understand them just by looking at them. Some of them are very obscure and hard to appreciate.

AA doesn't have a three thousand year tradition to call upon, but we can borrow wisdom from any source. These next sections offer useful, borrowed gems that can improve an alcoholic's life. Remember that by growing we don't lose anything except the shackles of alcoholism.

Stay away from one drink, one day at a time

This is a concept that we probably encountered at our first meeting. To remain sober all we need to do is to stay away from our first drink on a daily basis. If we don't take the first then the second and subsequent drinks cannot occur. We often challenge this idea. We argue that if we accept that we have an incurable illness and that drinking again is insanity, why not simply stop forever. This is yet another symptom of our illness. We seek to argue and impress when we should simply accept. We plan never to drink again and we are going to do this by not drinking one day at a time.

I was a few months away from my last drink driving down one of those long straight roads that go on into the distance forever. My mind suddenly said, "That is your life, on and on, Christmas, Holidays and Deaths all without a drink". Shaken, I knew that I couldn't face the idea. What would I do when faced

*with the death of my parents or a friend? There was absolutely
no point in continuing trying to stay away from drink because I
could see that I couldn't do it.*

*In the midst of this desolation echoed the suggestion that I had
heard at the meetings: Stay away from it for the rest of the day
and make a new decision tomorrow. My spirits lifted as this
finally made sense. I knew that I might decide to drink again,
but it wasn't going to be today.*

Instead of attempting the unachievable ideal of stopping
forever, we can manage the smaller and more achievable
decision – not to drink today. At first, it can prove too
difficult to achieve one day, but we can break it down
further and not drink for the next hour, after which we can
reassess the benefit of drinking. If during the hour, we
take positive action to help ourselves we will stay safe.

In layman terms, alcohol is rich in sugar and energy, when
our body feels starved and wants feeding it will trigger a
craving. Due to habit and the illness, our first reaction is to
assume that we need a drink. Because we have always
justified or rationalised our feelings, we genuinely might
not understand what people are talking about in
"craving". We have been thirsty and when we felt like a
drink, we took one. The cravings are insidious. They are
the hinted suggestion that a drink would be nice, if
ignored, they return in another guise- possibly that we
deserve a drink. They escalate until a drink is absolutely
the only thing that will enable us to survive. If we give in
to the first urge, we never experience the escalation and
consequently don't recognise the process.

There is no scientific support for the following simple
pieces of wisdom, but we can claim proof that they work.

Talking to another alcoholic is something we usually find
difficult. No matter how alien it is to us, this technique has

stood the test of time. A phrase like "a problem shared is a problem halved," would not exist if it had never worked. It is almost certain that we will reduce or remove a problem if we pick up the phone and talk to another person.

Taking a drink with some sugar in it, in this health conscious world, how we recoil from such a suggestion. We drank liquid that could run a rocket engine, but now object to added sugar. We were on a route to certain death, but we don't want to put on weight.

A pocket full of sweets can save the life of an alcoholic embarking on recovery. There can be no excuses for us. The illness is going to use its considerable cunning to trick us into taking a drink. By convincing us to ridicule the idea, we leave ourselves open to attack. We can actually feel self-conscious buying sweets, but this is simply the illness fighting back.

Changing our habits is essential, trying to behave exactly as we always have, except not drinking, doesn't work and can cause "drinking thinking". If we drank at a particular time, or with certain friends we can be tempted to switch to soft drinks and carry on doing this.

When I stopped drinking, I carried on meeting my friends, but switched to ordering tomato juice. One bottle was merely a mouthful compared to the beer I used to consume and I quickly escalated to having four in a glass. It was a bit of a joke, but my friends accepted this. Then one night as the barmaid served me she laughed and said, "Why don't you just get a tin of soup and a straw". I was furious and immediately ordered a beer…

Even if we don't drink, we can feel uneasy. Instead of perpetuating the same behaviour, it is better to throw ourselves out of our routine with something different, like taking some exercise or visiting a library.

Denial, denial, denial

Denial is such an intrinsic part of alcoholism we call it "the illness of denial". We deny that we have a problem or argue that the problem is everybody else's to deal with. We only had a drink because we were bored, lonely, tired, angry etc. Our family and friends continue the denial. They prefer to justify our behaviour rather than recognise that we are in the grip of an illness such as alcoholism.

A friend used his mother's denial of his illness to obtain alcohol. He had returned to his mother with a tale that his wife was refusing to let him drink the strong dark beer that kept him healthy. His mother saw her fearful and weak son and wanted to help him. She was over eighty and could only walk with the aid of a frame, but every day she went to the shops to buy his "medicine". His wife pleaded with his mother to stop, but she could see how much her son improved when he had his beer and continued until he died.

Even in recovery, we continue to deny how much the monkey and our own self-will influences our motives. We are the masters of justification and learning to be honest about our behaviour is the part of living sober that eventually means people will trust what we are saying. Only by recognising that we are denying the full extent of the sickness, do we really come to terms with it and start to recover. Certainly, in the early days this is characterised by the phrase:

I can't be an alcoholic because...

- My friends drink more than I ever did.

- A glass of wine is good for circulation and I only drink wine.

- Alcoholics drink all the time and I only drink at the

184

weekend.

I still look back bemused at my first contact with AA. To me, appearance was everything and so the house was tidy, I wore expensive clothes and thought I looked great. I couldn't see the overall impression, like an invalid, I sat propped up in a chair, wasted and frail with my feet bloated and my skin a sickly grey. I listened, but they seemed to be talking nonsense when they talked about dying. My own "I can't be because" was that because I hadn't had an alcoholic fit for nearly a year I was getting better. It was only a matter of time before I recovered fully. I wished them well and they left.

HALT – Danger Sign (Hungry Angry Lonely Tired)

It is worth thinking of these as the younger brothers of the four horsemen of the apocalypse. When we experience one, the rest usually appear. Their arrival heralds a "brain storm" of dangerous thinking, but they are magical and travel in disguise. Regardless of length of sobriety, we insist that "people, places or things" are the problem and fail to recognise the true cause of our feelings.

I am certain that my mouth dropped open when I heard this at my first meeting and I thought somebody must have told them how I lived my life. I was always late in the morning and rushed out without eating anything. I lived in constant conflict with the fools that I had to work with leaving me angry and isolated from them. To make up for their incompetence I worked through my lunch break and long into the evening. I finished my day by grabbing an instant meal of some form and drowning the day out with drink. The idea of eliminating these stresses from my life seemed more difficult than stopping drinking.

We rarely manage to avoid them completely. We all choose to skip lunch or to put more into the day than we can cope with. When we are having a difficult time, it is worth running a quick check. Mentally say, "HALT" and see if we are suffering the aftermath of allowing them to occur. We can usually laugh at our own stupidity and see that there is nothing wrong that a chat and a sandwich won't cure.

Going back to basics

People say this at meetings as if they had progressed to some higher level of the program. They confess that life has become too difficult and they are correcting the drift by "going back to basics". There is no higher level, there are only basics and of course, we should go back to them.

I had been lucky that my company had supported me when I needed to take a few months off with "stress". They weren't aware that I had attended my first AA meeting and after a faltering start had discovered I was an alcoholic.

In school, I had always excelled at study and exams and thought the AA program was just another test I had to revise for and pass. I followed the suggestions, read the books and soon felt able to return to work. My company allowed me to ease myself back in part time, but I quickly returned to running most of the department. As I did this, I found that "living in the day" and the other sayings didn't help during my hectic working day. The demands of work conflicted with my regular meetings and if I prayed at all, it was in the car on the way to the office.

I lasted six months before my wife found me sitting in the car on the driveway long after I had left the house. I took the day off and spoke with a few friends from AA. That evening I was at a meeting and shared what I had been doing. It seemed too simple, but all I could do was to hope to return to the basics of the program that had put me on my feet in the first place.

Correcting ourselves after realising we have drifted is how

most of us progress and there is nothing wrong with acknowledging that we need to return to the principles of the program. Our old life was our comfort zone for a long time and to expect to change, never to drift back into old behaviour would be unrealistic.

Accept that alcoholism is an illness

A memory haunts me. I remember that even though I had told her not to, my wife had gone out and left me in charge of getting our children ready for bed. I was annoyed with her because I had been working all day and wanted to unwind. I put the children in the bath, squirted them with washing up liquid and went downstairs. I put on some loud music and opened a bottle. I intended to relax even if she was determined that I wouldn't.

After a few more beers, I heard a small voice from the top of the stairs, "Dad, can we get out, we are all blue and crinkly". I ran up the stairs shaking my fist screaming at them. I couldn't believe they had the nerve to disturb me. The look of fear on my son's face is etched into my memory. He stood trembling and crying whilst I raged at them.

When I embarked upon recovery, I could not conceive how I would ever be able to live with the memory of creating such pain in their young lives.

Grasping the fact that alcoholism is an illness is an important step towards accepting a recovery. If we believe alcoholism is an illness, we understand the statement, "can you feel guilty about having spots when you catch measles". Clinicians worldwide recognise it, but we still argue that this isn't true. Who are we to argue against these people? The answer of course is that we are alcoholic and regardless of the facts, arrogant enough to argue against anybody and anything.

Whilst accepting it as an illness frees us from guilt

concerning our actions before we knew we had it. It makes us responsible, regardless of the justification, for not re-activating our behaviour.

We can no longer shrug our shoulders and ignore the consequences of the decision to drink. We know that to drink is to descend into insanity. More than that, as we work through our defects, we realise we cannot hide behind the belief that the only person we hurt is ourselves.

Never test sobriety

This doesn't mean doing things like holding a drink close to our mouth and not drinking it. There are many ways we "test" our sobriety, dramatically declaring, "If this doesn't stop I will end up drinking again," admits the possibility of drinking being an option.

We sometimes try to apply conditions regarding sobriety as motivational goals. We insist that we will stay sober if we manage to regain our partner and family. It seems tempting to use this kind of trick as encouragement, but they can only work for a short time and if the condition succeeds or fails, what do we do then?

Here are a few examples of other ways we test our sobriety:

• Going too long without meetings

• Pushing the boundaries of honest living a bit too far

• Becoming too proud to share openly about a difficulty

• Wandering aimlessly up the drinks aisle at the supermarket

It had always been my Saturday lunchtime routine to go to the corner shop. I would buy a loaf of bread, cigarettes, a lottery ticket and a half bottle of rum. When I started trying to get sober, I simply kept to the same routine, but didn't buy the rum. I talked to somebody at the meeting and they suggested that I was "testing my sobriety" by needlessly shopping where I could buy drink. I thought they were being silly, especially when my local shop is so handy.

One particular weekend I was upset. My son was supposed to be coming home and I had been looking forward to the visit. He called and said that something had come up and he couldn't make the journey. I had wanted him to see how much I had improved after my short time not drinking. I went to the corner shop and I don't remember buying the rum, but it was there when I got home. I knew I shouldn't leave it on the kitchen table, but I also knew that I was going to be on my own for the whole weekend and nobody would know if I drank it. It was open and half-empty before I even thought about it. It took many months to pluck up the courage to go back to the meeting and confess how stupid I had been.

Don't make any major decisions for the first two years

We are all told this, but rarely believe it. It is only after we have lived through the first two years that we can see what a great piece of advice it is and start to "pass it on" to newcomers ourselves. At the two-year point, we look back and see that we had been functioning with the emotional stability of a two year old on food additives. We also accept that we are probably still not as stable as we had once imagined and continue to avoid making important decisions for ourselves. Whilst most of us ignore this advice, somebody occasionally listens, or at least gains a momentary pause in a headlong spiral into an avoidable disaster.

When I finally accepted defeat and came to my first meeting, I knew that my real problem was my husband. He was a pig and anybody who had to live with him would drink. All of my other friends had agreed with me that he was a burden and I was a little surprised that the women in the group didn't understand what I was telling them. Instead, they just kept saying, "stop drinking and keep coming to meetings."

As the days turned into weeks and months, I was still convinced that I would have to get divorced from him before I would be able to enjoy a full life again. The people at the meeting kept smiling and telling me to wait for two years before I did anything. I didn't notice the point at which he changed, but it was some time after I had stopped drinking and started to work through the program. I realised that he wasn't always wrong and actually had some well-buried feelings. I then found that we enjoyed life together and I couldn't remember what was so difficult to live with. I now feel that I was blaming all of my defects on him and that by working on removing them from me, I removed them from him as well.

Inventory Taking (of others)

Inventory taking is possibly one of the most subtle weapons the monkey can use against us. It is a worthless thief of time and peace of mind. We could be enjoying life, but instead we become transfixed by the perceived wrongdoing of others. This is not the healthy inventory taking of step four, this is when we look at other people and judge what they should or should not be doing. We usually first hear that we should not take other people's inventories when we are critical of somebody at a meeting and it is a common mistake to believe that this instruction only applies within AA. It can take a long time before we come to realise that we seem to live our lives by continually judging everything from individuals up to major international corporations.

My ex-wife had always been a bit unstable – after all, she married me when I was drinking. We had a daughter, but we separated and I didn't see either of them for quite a long time.

When I started to have contact again, I found myself drawn into their arguments. My daughter told me of her mother's behaviour and I was frustrated that she had to survive in such a damaging home life. My ex-wife told me of our daughter's tantrums. I felt trapped in the middle as I watched them throw stones at each other. My time became absorbed in the attempt to reconcile them, dragging me down until it suddenly struck me how helpless I was. All I was witnessing was their relationship and I was entirely powerless to intervene.

At times, they still draw me into their world of tantrums and accusations and I have yet to benefit from my involvement. I am sure they are wrong, but it is not mine to judge. They seem to need this friction to survive. Maybe one day I will be able to accept it.

We never take inventory in a constructive fashion inspiring us into positive action. *Our contentment is inversely proportional to the amount of time we spend judging how other people are behaving.*

Never say - At my stage in sobriety

This phrase will cross all of our minds during our recovery. Initially, we possibly cannot imagine how we would ever try to cope with a problem without the support of the group or our sponsor, but it is almost certain that we will feel this way at some time. The monkey traps us with it and prevents us from sharing honestly. We encounter a problem that we believe we should be able to handle and feel unable to reveal it in case people laugh at us.

I was over ten years sober when they asked me to join the golf club committee. This meant that I could not get to my home group every week as the meetings coincided, but I was confident that this was not going to be a problem and I knew I could make a real difference to the way the club was running.

The stupidity of these people stunned me. At every committee meeting, I had to lose my temper before they would listen. I knew this was not "sober" behaviour, but it seemed to be the only way to manage them. I remember thinking "At my time in sobriety I should be able to cope with these people".

My frustration spilled over into my home life and I noticed that my whole family were also stupid and I had to shout at them constantly. Finally, this frustration came with me to an AA meeting and I ended up hurting somebody I thought needed putting back on track. Outside the meeting, my sponsor spoke to me and enquired about what I had been doing. He "suggested" that I had my priorities wrong and that I might not be up to taking on the battles of the golf world. Although it hurt to give up the committee, I went along with the suggestion. Incredibly quickly, the people in AA stopped being stupid and so did my family. I don't know about the golf committee, today I just play golf there.

We have become proud of our sobriety and don't want to go to the meeting and confess that something as simple as life has thrown us. We certainly don't want to risk somebody coming up to us and giving us advice about how to cope with the problem. It is essential that we recognise and laugh at the thought as soon as it comes into our head. *Learning to laugh at our own pomposity removes another of the weapons from the hands of the monkey and helps us to understand humility.*

Confusion

Regardless of how long we have been sober, we can confuse ourselves by comparing our life against how we imagine other people live. At times, everybody seems to be enjoying life more than we do and we become disenchanted with our sobriety.

Is there a better way? Private Clinics and Counselling

Nobody can get another person sober. If they could, our families and partners would have succeeded. We need to reach the point where we take responsibility for our own recovery, because until we recognise our excuses for what they are, we believe the problem is everybody else's.

A person sent to a private clinic often thinks that somebody else is going to do the hard work. They might stop drinking by remaining in a restrictive environment and even start out with an honest desire to get well, but at some point this switches into "I got away with it again" and the rest of the treatment becomes a game. Group sessions become an opportunity to be melodramatic and counsellors are there to bait. The alcoholic delights in leading the counsellor smugly towards the answers they choose to expose, possibly believing that it gives a display of superior intellect and cunning. It is common to feel that a counsellor who cannot see through our obvious deceptions is useless. Whatever the reason, until we accept defeat, there seems little permanent value in expensive treatment.

Many people who have been to private clinics do now lead successful lives within AA. Nobody has to pay to adopt the program, but sometimes we value something more if we do. Undeniably, attending a private clinic can give a person a flying start, rather like taking an intensive driving course to learn how to drive. Exactly like the driving course, we gain the basic skills, but the wider experience required to survive can only come with time.

Our chance of success doesn't seem dependent upon starting in a clinic or at AA. When we come out of the clinic we must practice the program exactly the same way as the person who started by making a call to the AA helpline and attending meetings.

Opinions

Opinions – Giving ours

In the bar room people are willing to offer their opinion on just about any topic and they require little genuine knowledge of the subject. This isn't just alcoholics, most people try to offer helpful suggestions and the temptation to give opinions is extremely strong.

Within AA, we encounter people at various stages of alcoholism, all capable of coping with different things. We don't recover at the same rate and we don't have the same resilience. Our well-meaning opinion has the power to kill another alcoholic and we should only offer it sparingly. Thoughtless remarks can cause problems, even when we think the topic isn't part of their alcoholism. We might make a "helpful" comment regarding their choice of car, place they live or the people they live with. We usually offer little but disharmony when we comment on other people's way of life and we need to learn to keep our opinion to ourselves.

Opinions – listening to others

I had been coming to meetings for a few months when my husband left. I felt that my world had ended and although I didn't want to drink, the pressure was becoming too great to handle.

I went to the doctor and he prescribed some tablets that calmed me down and allowed me to get on with life. I was much better and I shared this at my home group. After the meeting a woman came up to me and aggressively told me that I should flush them down the toilet because I was simply taking my booze in a solid form and that I would drink again if I continued to use them.

Each week this woman came up to me, narrowed her eyes and scornfully asked if I was still taking them. I felt belittled and undermined, I started to believe that I would only be able to achieve sobriety once I was not taking anything.

Thankfully, my sponsor told me that I should take medical advice from a doctor and rarely from other alcoholics. After a short time, my doctor took me off the tablets in a controlled way and I was able to live my life without them.

It is amazing how many people have dangerous opinions. We will encounter people with forceful advice about "the correct route". Somebody who feels they know best can challenge any facet of our life, religion, drugs, relationships, work etc. A correct decision is to listen to what these people have to say and then to take their comments to somebody who knows us to see if the "suggestion" was appropriate.

Outside AA, we will encounter complete strangers who will dismissively question our decision to stop drinking. By allowing others to voice their negative opinion, we are opening our minds to the possibility that we were wrong. Suddenly, it seems likely that we had only been "going through a bad patch" and now that our life is settled, we no longer need to continue. Sometimes people want us to start drinking again because our abstinence emphasises their drinking. Others think that they are being helpful, or showing off their intellect. Some people just need to sneer at what others consider important.

The program can seem too simple and we yearn for something more substantial to fix our problems. Paradoxically, the program can seem too difficult and we don't want to follow it. At times of doubt, the monkey seems able to guide us towards people brimming over with good advice and confusing opinions. It is important to recognise these situations and evaluate what has given this person such an insight into our condition that they can diagnose and correct what others cannot.

Opinions – of the stars

The worst kind of distraction is possibly the celebrity drunk. The problem with celebrities is that they have access to the media. They go on television and give interviews that appear worldwide in magazines and newspapers. How many people justify continuing to drink by comparing their behaviour to that of a celebrity drunk?

I recall watching Oliver Reed in a drunken state on a chat show and thinking "yes! That's the lifestyle I want, I want to behave wild and unfettered." There were some things missing that prevented me from fully adopting his way of life, such as money, fame, acting talent etc. However, I had managed to become bloated and unacceptably loud and this seemed a good start.

Many of us are bursting with enthusiasm when we realise that life is not ending and that we are going to recover. We can be over-zealous for a time, having "found AA", we want to evangelise and recruit others into our new way of life. Luckily, most of us can only reach a relatively low number of people. This is not true for the celebrity in early recovery and many of them choose to shout from the rooftops, "I'm in AA". Doing this they are holding themselves up to scrutiny. If they don't stay sober, their marriage fails, or indeed, they do anything, people judge them and AA. The monkey on our shoulder is waiting to whisper its own judgement, "That AA thing doesn't work, look at them, with their money and fame they failed, what is the point in trying?"

Some celebrities have recovered using a twelve-step program, but now publicly disparage what it can do. These belittling comments tend to take the form of "I went whilst I had a problem, but don't go any more because..." citing religion, God or other commitments. This can damage other people in two ways. Firstly, it may encourage somebody who is struggling into drinking again. Secondly, our family can think that if "Mr. X" has recovered and no longer needs to go to meetings, then we shouldn't either.

Whilst others may try to tempt us from our path to recovery, the celebrity knows how to deliver a line. Whether we like it or not they have a lot of power over our thinking and avoiding the distraction created by celebrities is an important lesson to learn.

We can quietly admire those celebrities where it is common knowledge that they are members, but who do not publicly discuss it. We should feel compassion for those who appear on the chat show proclaiming a cure after a couple of meetings. If they fail, they will fall harder than the normal person will. Finally, remember that celebrity status rarely requires intelligence and humility. Who should we trust, the quiet chap at the meeting with thirty years sobriety, or a fading star?

A new set of emotions

Alcoholics are often emotionally immature. We behave as if we "stalled" our emotional growth at the age that we started to drink. Whilst we are drinking, we rarely question our reactions. Like a petulant adolescent, our behaviour, beliefs, and feelings are unquestionably correct. When we stop drinking, our emotions start to come back to life and we find ourselves plagued by strange feelings that we have never acknowledged before.

Some emotions share the names of the defects that we are trying to avoid like, pride, anger and envy or the positive virtues like charity and compassion. These are primitive and powerful forces within our lives. Other emotions such as, confused, melancholy, cheated and lonely can be more difficult to identify. All of these feelings combine to motivate us in some way.

I feel that when I was drinking I didn't actually have any emotions. I faked them to get an effect. I would say, "I love you" to get somebody to say it back to me, or I would scream and rage to make somebody do what I wanted. Even many years into sobriety I envy people who can move through a whole range of appropriate emotions where I find myself hampered by anger and insecurities with an on/ off switch.

Not on the list of defects

Sometimes we drift away from sober thinking, but we don't see the behaviour as defective because our specific problem doesn't appear to be on the "standard list" of defects.

I noticed that I wasn't going to be able to pay off my credit card,

it had been an expensive month and I had treated myself to a
new computer. The next month my car needed some work and I
had to buy a new printer. Then the washing machine broke down
and I needed a new one. I realised I was getting deeper in trouble
and I was feeling uneasy. I checked my behaviour, pride, greed,
envy, etc. All of my expenditure was necessary, I hadn't wanted
to show off my washing machine and I certainly hadn't bought
things to compete with next door.

The snowball of moving debt between credit cards bounced out
of control as increasingly threatening letters started to arrive
from debt collection services. All I had wanted was a
comfortable, peaceful sobriety, but I was now living in a misery
of confusion that seemed to be pushing me towards drinking.

A defect is behaviour that damages anybody - including
us. When we recognise our behaviour as harmful, our first
efforts should go into changing. Possibly, somebody else
could interpret our actions within a framework of "named
defects", but we are not playing "swords and sorcery"
riddles and learning the name of the demon doesn't
necessarily reduce its strength. Part of deciding how to
change is to describe how we are feeling to somebody else.
The important part is clearly identifying what we are
doing wrong and it doesn't matter if it takes one or one
hundred words to describe the feelings.

Making up for lost time

Initially, we are comfortable with the idea that we need to
be good to ourselves. We are willing to accept that we
aren't "materially wealthy," but we are happy that we are
becoming "spiritually wealthy". As time passes, the lustre
wears off our spiritual wealth and we become tempted
into rejoining the rat race. When the phrase "I didn't get
sober to…" is used, we are usually justifying something
that isn't in our best interest.

Regardless of the warnings, the monkey tricks us into taking inventories again. We gaze enviously at the house or car our friend has acquired, feeling that we deserve similar luxuries. Resentment drives us into trying to achieve more than is sensible, creating the conditions where sobriety loses its priority.

We abandon our spiritual development by focusing upon material desires. If we look at this style of thinking and then refer back to the major defects we discussed earlier, pride, envy, greed, lust and anger, we will find that we are experiencing most, if not all of these defects. There is nothing wrong with aspiring to improve our future situation, providing we don't compromise our sobriety trying to achieve it.

Challenges

Life goes on and continues to put obstacles in our way. Challenges are how we learn. If survival had been too easy, the human race wouldn't have evolved. Presented with a challenge, we try to use our reasoning capacity to decide upon a correct solution. Quick fixes are rarely the answer and we should always question our "good ideas", is it the monkey or us?

Drugs

The protective cocoon of alcohol means that we rarely have to face the realities of life and the thought of living without any form of support frightens us. Alcohol changes our mood on demand and we become unable to manage our feelings naturally. Scared, we look for other chemicals to help us, ignoring the fact that these are as destructive and addictive as the drink we are trying to avoid.

There is nothing wrong with using medicine as prescribed, but any form of drug can be abused, Recreational, Prescription or Patent. Possibly as many alcoholics have damaged their sobriety with cough medicine as have with cannabis. At three in the morning, a small dose of cough syrup can seem similar to a shot of rum and the thought that they are really the same can lead us back into drinking.

As well as those of us tempted to use drugs after stopping drinking, there are also many alcoholics with the dual problem of drug and alcohol abuse. In virtually every case, they decide to carry on using drugs whilst giving up drinking. Some manage to do so successfully, but in most cases, they say that they didn't experience a good sobriety until they gave up using drugs as well.

We trigger old behaviour by revisiting old situations. Acquiring recreational drugs possibly means coming into contact with people that we would be better off avoiding. We are not trying to become saints, but the monkey is always waiting for the opportunity to tempt us. Chemically changing our emotions creates a fertile situation for temptation to occur. When we deliberately lower our inhibitions, we invite the monkey to lead us gradually away from sobriety and it isn't long before the suggestion of a drink starts to occur.

Perfection – Surely, that is what is expected!

It is hard to imagine somebody walking past the house of a drinking alcoholic saying, "That's the house of a perfectionist!" In the later stages of our drinking, the lawn remains uncut for months, the window frames need to be painted and we rarely open the curtains. We think that we are perfectionists, but we are blind to the incongruous realities around us.

Perfectionism cripples us. When we realise that we cannot be the best at something, we give up. If we take an exam with an eighty percent pass mark, we think anything less than one hundred percent is a failure and we become disheartened. For some reason our best is never good enough. We imagine that we are on a pedestal and always expected to succeed, torturing ourselves with a fear of failure and the thought of people seeing us fail. Nobody expects total infallibility from other people and if they do, it is highlighting their problems rather than ours.

Step One is the only thing we have to get completely right. We have to be convinced that we are powerless over alcohol – and that our lives had become unmanageable. Any time we stray from the fundamental starting point, the monkey awakens and life descends into chaos.

Suffering from minor ailments

Colds and flu often raise the accusation that men are pathetic when they are suffering, whereas women soldier on. Regardless of gender, alcoholics act irrationally when they are ill. Our thinking seems affected in direct relationship to our rising temperature, and we suddenly feel the need to make major changes to our lives. If we can bring ourselves to talk to somebody, they will listen and laugh, telling us that we are ill and shouldn't make any decisions. Although this seems simple and logical when we feel healthy, it is surprisingly difficult to accept when we have streaming eyes and realise that we MUST address a major life problem.

Dieting and Smoking

It is dangerous to try to address problems like weight and smoking in the first couple of years. The cravings triggered by either of these can easily be mistaken for a need to drink and distract us from our primary focus – to stay sober.

We rarely have the patience to follow a slow, sensible diet. We want quick solutions such as pills that magically make weight drop away. These pills work by increasing our metabolism and producing a "high". Whilst other people cope with this, we should view any chemical that changes how we feel with caution. We can misread the mood swings as something more sinister, or if we are bursting with energy, we are tempted to double the dose to feel even better.

Smoking is an addiction and although some people manage to stop by using the twelve-step program, many don't. Discovering how difficult it is to stop smoking shocks us, we believed that our toughest battle had been to stop drinking and that anything else would be easy. The mental upheavals created by stopping smoking are different to those we experience when we stop drinking. Dramatic emotional swings and physical craving can plague us for many months, but we fail to recognise them for what they are. We can feel angry, depressed, or lethargic and the monkey uses these feelings to push us off the path of recovery.

If we try to diet or stop smoking, we are usually far more successful if we take advice and instruction, rather than deciding to invent our own way. Changing our behaviour always awakens the monkey and we open the door to the major character defects we thought we had addressed.

Pride can make us look for attention and compliments. If they don't come, we are disappointed and if they do, we can become "intoxicated" by the fuss somebody makes of us.

Intolerance creeps in as we sneer piously when others fail to achieve what we have been able to do.

Low self-esteem can emerge if we fail to achieve the goal we set for ourselves.

Getting honest about our illness with other people

When we stop drinking, we change. If we live with a partner, we are hurt when they don't "read our minds". Instead of knowing what we expect of them, they carry on, apparently showing little concern regarding our sobriety. If we don't acknowledge our illness, our partners will expect us to live the same life we always have done. If we don't tell them, they won't know that we are uncomfortable around drunks and drink, after all, it never used to bother us.

Regardless of whether our partner lived with us through our dark times or has come along later, we need to discuss our problems concerning drink and drinking situations with them. Without doing so, we are allowing the monkey to confuse us with the sayings that we hear at meetings, "We cannot change anybody but ourselves" or "Strong sobriety can be maintained under any conditions". Both of which are true when placed in context, but are not particularly relevant to this aspect of our lives.

We can be tempted into trying to adopt a double life and behave differently when we are amongst our old friends to the way we behave when we are with other alcoholics. There are a few reasons why we would do this:

Leaving a doorway back is one of the common reasons. If we don't tell people that we are trying to change, they won't criticise us if we fail or interfere if we decide to drink.

The idea of anonymity can confuse us. We know that "what we hear in the room – stays in the room", but we take this suggestion too far. This should be true about the detail of who, where and what, but not the underlying principles.

Making up for past behaviour seems attractive. We trick ourselves into staying quiet and we can pretend that we are starting working on our ninth step.

Avoiding confrontation can mean that we don't speak out when we should do. We can be frightened of confrontation, or scared of the emotional backlash we feel when we do confront a difficult problem.

What actually happens is that instead of calmly discussing our problem, we unexpectedly explode. We unleash a verbal tirade at our loved one. We tell them that they are lacking in consideration and how much support we expect from them. These irrational explosions confuse our family and damage the trust that we have been building up. Honesty means that we don't use our alcoholism like a club to bully our partners, but we don't surrender our rights either, ending up resentful about doing so.

Becoming the convenient driver

We don't usually mind being the driver, we know that we are going to be with people who have been drinking, but we rationalise that because we are sober and working our program, we will be able to cope. Part of our defence strategy for drinking situations is that we should have an escape route planned, but agreeing to drive traps us. We will have to wait until people are ready to leave or abandon them. Either decision can be the cause of conflict and stress.

Drunks are unpredictable and unconcerned with our discomfort. Any time drink is involved, we should question our motives. Are we being sensible and helpful, or are we putting ourselves at risk? Are we "fishing" for compliments from the other people, hoping to draw attention to our sobriety? Driving a car full of drunks can be stressful and we can feel isolated. Possibly, we are thoughtlessly allowing Hungry, Angry, Lonely, and Tired (HALT) into our life. When we are honest about our motives and think things through, we can make a decision and act appropriately. We can agree to drive, but we should not allow others to assume that we will always do so. By discussing the situation, we are humbly accepting our vulnerability, rather than testing our sobriety.

Drink around the home

One of the first trials we encounter when we stop drinking is getting rid of the booze around us. We usually arranged things so that we had easy access to drink, ranging from a pack of beer in the corner through to prominently displayed crystal decanters. We think that it is essential to our home and feel that our partner would object if we removed them from view.

A recovering alcoholic has no valid excuse to have alcohol in the house, our partner does, but failing to discuss the fact that it make us uneasy is "testing our sobriety". We could take the view that tipping their bottle of twenty five year old brandy down the sink will teach them, or we could be less confrontational and simply ask them to keep it out of sight.

Why would somebody refuse a reasonable request?

Unwilling to listen, when we first try to stop drinking, they might no longer be the "loving partner" that we thought they were. Our behaviour as a practicing alcoholic damages people and they may be unable to listen to our pleas. If this is the case, only time will regain their trust and we merely harden their resolve against us if we try to demand support.

Losing their "drinking buddy", if our relationship started when our drinking wasn't an apparent problem, they can be frightened that we will change too much and no longer be a part of their life.

Saving us from another crazy obsession often motivates our partners into failing to support us. They have lived through us chasing various "cures" and they are scared that we will become lost in "happy clappy" behaviour.

Simply not understanding is the most common reason for other people not helping us. We openly discuss our feelings with people outside our home, but fail to do so with the people who live with us.

When I first got sober, my daughter would have friends around for the evening. They would leave a half-empty bottle of wine in the fridge and unwashed glasses around in the lounge. I didn't complain because I felt that my "motherly" behaviour in the past had been non-existent and I thought I was establishing a Mother / Daughter relationship.

One night when I couldn't sleep, I opened the fridge door looking for milk and found a bottle of wine. My mind instantly ran through all of the facts. It was late and nobody would know if I drank it. Excuses flooded in, "It wasn't my fault I had been taken by surprise", "I was half asleep – virtually sleep walking". I immediately started working out how I would be able to get another bottle - did I have the money and where could I buy it. I had changed from justifying an accidental drink into planning the next one in less than a second.

I didn't drink, but the next day I had a long discussion with my daughter. She hadn't even thought about what she was doing because she had grown up with bottles of wine in the fridge. I still find the odd glass lurking where a friend has put it down by the side of a chair, but things have improved dramatically.

Like any change, there will be times when it slips from the other person's attention. We shouldn't be discouraged and give up the first time somebody forgets. This isn't just an "early days" problem, our families grow up and our partners change. The bottom line is that it is our responsibility to keep ourselves safe and failing to be honest can easily evolve into an "at my time in sobriety" trap.

Tricks to help

The art of constructive removal

We often hear the word *Serenity* within AA and many
meetings close using the "serenity prayer".

> *God grant me the*
> *Serenity to accept the things I cannot change*
> *Courage to change the things I can*
> *And Wisdom to know the difference*

Most of us recognise that life will improve if we fulfil each
line. The lines are also in the correct sequence. Without
attaining serenity, our chances of achieving the remaining
ideals are doubtful. Our courage is more likely to be
bluster and our wisdom merely self-will.

Our first experiences of serenity flash like a fluorescent
tube flickering in a dark tunnel, there and then gone. We
cannot demand serenity, but we can achieve it by
removing its opposites. Serenity is like a pathway through
a desert; always present, but often covered by sand blown
across it. To find the path we have to uncover it. To
maintain it, we have to keep clearing away the sand that
constantly tries to hide it again.

Western society drives us to acquire things to make us
happy, a better house, more money, expensive clothes. The
program encourages us to acquire positive virtues, we
want to increase our humility, gain acceptance and rely
upon a Higher Power. In the same way that we can get
more serenity by removing things, we can increase
humility, by reducing pride and increase acceptance by
reducing expectation.

This is not a spiritual philosophy but a balance
demonstrated in many ways. A motorcycle can go faster

either by increasing the power of the engine, or by making the motorcycle lighter. A business becomes more profitable either by increasing sales, or by reducing costs - taking away is just as effective as adding to.

A common cliché is, "you can't find God, because he isn't lost", a true, but useless statement. We find our keys by removing the coat that was on top of them, somebody helpfully telling us they were always there serves no purpose. Finding a Higher Power by removing obstacles is the same, it was always there, but obscured. More appropriate guidance would be that we shouldn't *frantically search* for a Higher Power by desperately adopting different religions, sects or beliefs in the hope that we will become spiritual.

To improve our life, we <u>might</u> find that the answer is to stop doing something, rather than to start doing something.

Toolkit for normal living

Is one way to describe the program, but before a toolkit can be of any use, we have learn which tool to use for a specific task. We could use either a hammer or a screwdriver to dismantle a clock, but only a screwdriver is appropriate if we want it to work again.

When we realise that turmoil has replaced serenity and life has descended into chaos, we can use the program to help us identify the problem. A good way to do this is to work backwards through the steps to see if they contain a solution. It seems easier to challenge ourselves by working down, rather than up and it is more effective if we do this with a friend or sponsor. Once we have identified where our behaviour is awry we can work out a plan to correct it.

Have we put out our hand to anybody? Even when we don't want to, getting involved with other people is an essential part of our recovery. We trick ourselves by thinking that we will do more harm than good in our "fragile" state, but this is exactly the time when we should have the humility to speak to other people.

Are we allowing enough time to improve our conscious contact? It is easy to allow normal life to eat away at our time and start to rely on our own inner, rather than outer resources.

Should we be acknowledging recent behaviour as part of our inventory? We can fall back into our old ways of dealing with people, especially when we become determined to achieve an important goal. We can also find that we are exhibiting entirely new forms of defective behaviour. The tricks we encounter are endless and without a regular review, old and new defects are certain to emerge.

Do we have unfulfilled amends that are causing a problem?

Our life moves on and we drift in and out of contact with people. Somebody unexpectedly coming out of our past can uncover forgotten situations and reveal additional amends we owe.

Are we allowing our defects to drive our actions? We have to look and decide if pride, greed, envy etc. is the real reason behind decisions that we have recently made. Are we still living with a defect we actively sought to have removed? Are we coming to the point where a "second crop" defect is now becoming apparent?

Is self-will motivating our actions? Few manage to hand their will and their life over and not snatch it back. In normal life the fine line between could and should is a decision that we can get wrong. *Moral behaviour isn't necessarily what we do, but often what we refrain from doing.*

Is our current action insane? We can often look back and recognise insanity within actions that we have justified as sane an hour earlier.

Do we believe that a Higher Power could restore us to sanity? Do we really trust a Higher Power or merely pay lip service to the idea? It can be easy to put our heads down and continue with something even through we can see that we are acting irrationally. We know that we have a faith in a Higher Power, but we don't want to risk our HP getting it wrong and failing to make the correct decision.

Have we been trying to control things we have no control over? We can become frustrated with the taxman, the weather or anything that affects us. Our "right" to do what we want to do can blind us to the reality of the situation we are facing.

How much time have we spent around drink? Drinking

situations damage our thinking on many subtle levels and although we can justify our actions, it is dangerous to spend too much time around drink.

We drift across a fine line, from acceptable into unacceptable. When the illness managed our life, we frequently and knowingly ignored the moral boundaries of society. We possibly enjoyed imagining the impression we created, although many say that they simply didn't recognise that rules applied to them.

If I needed to park my car, I parked, oblivious to the restriction sign. If I needed to be somewhere, I drove at the speed that would get me there, regardless of the limits. If I had been drinking, I would drive home. My car was essential to me, but I didn't recognise that flouting the law was risking my livelihood.

When I wanted "love", I picked somebody up. I didn't care about them or their life. When I needed cash, I took it from them. If they objected, I hit them – hard. I liked being different. I wasn't unfeeling - I just didn't see that I was wrong.

Living by the "rules" of society is living a "sober" life. We now recognise the existence of these boundaries, but when they constrict us, we need help adhering to them. Losing focus upon the principles embodied in the program means that Sobriety Lost Its Priority. A drink is the final confirmation of a "SLIP" not the first indication.

Also consider...

If it damages your sobriety give it up has to be one of the greatest double-edged swords handed to a newcomer. Whilst true, it provides a dangerously convenient excuse. We can construe just about any activity as damaging to our sobriety. Getting out of bed and going to work interrupts our quiet time for contemplation. Going to the supermarket for food can be stressful and potentially disturbing. Tolerating a partner who seems to be constantly demanding attention is surely damaging our serenity.

We should be willing to give up anything that is damaging our sobriety, but we are not always the correct person to judge a situation. Before we act, it is better to check these decisions with somebody we trust. They sometimes spot a significant flaw in our plan and keep us from harming ourselves or other people.

Letting go of the concrete lifebelt is a useful illustration how fixed opinions often prove to be a liability. The image is that life is like swimming across a lake and we are desperately hanging on to what we mistake as a lifebelt. Our lifebelt is actually made out of concrete and if we stopped to examine it, we would see that life would become easier if we could just let go.

Willing to go to any lengths to achieve sobriety is a statement we come across in early days. We nod our heads and say, "of course we are willing," then we realise that we have to change fundamental aspects of our life. We suddenly whittle down our professed willingness to go to any lengths into doing what the monkey suggests we can accept.

Our concrete life belts or unacceptable changes can be many things, such as no longer being a member of the darts team, or throwing away the booze sitting in the kitchen. We are horrified and claim that life will stop if we don't continue doing... The benefits of our new way of life will remain out of reach whilst we insist on keeping one foot in the past. Learn to let go and watch the concrete lifebelt sink down into the depths.

Write to ourselves

Sometimes when we carry too many things in our heads, we become confused and get them out of perspective. Communicating with another alcoholic is a good way to solve problems, but there are times when we can clear our thinking by putting things down on paper. Making lists is a good habit to develop, but like many good habits, it takes time to become part of us. When we are under pressure, the last thing we want to do is to stop and make a list. In reality, it is the first thing that we should do. Lists remove some of the stress from our lives by allowing us to become more organised. Once we get in the habit, we realise that we can work through far more than we anticipate and we stop forgetting important tasks.

List of things we want to do, we sometimes need to fill a few spare hours. We know that wasting them leaves us feeling that we have slipped back into old ways. If we have a handy list of things we want to do, we can give ourselves a surprise treat and feel much better about the way we have spent the time.

List of things we don't want to do, we all have tasks that we don't want to do but have to achieve. We cheer ourselves up and feel relieved when we get something done from this list.

Lists of tasks, by keeping our daily tasks under control we achieve more and avoid having last minute panics when we realise that we have not done something that we intended to do.

Lists of fears when we are feeling threatened and uneasy, it is good to put our fears down on paper. In our head, they surface like monsters from the deep, we see each of them clearly for a short time, but as one fades, another pushes forward to replace it. By taking them out of our head, we can see that they are not as overwhelming or numerous as we had thought and we can start to think about solutions rather than problems.

Check your meeting count.

How many meetings should we be doing after one year, two years or ten years? The simple answer is – sufficient. A good piece of advice is to get to as many as we possibly can. It is easy to drop meetings out of our weekly schedule, but it is difficult to squeeze them back in. If we drop a meeting, it is important to take careful stock as time passes. Are we really feeling ok and functioning as well as we had been doing? Alcoholism is a cunning, patient illness and pride can stand in the way of going back to meetings we have dropped.

Try a God Can

The first time I heard this idea, I was repulsed, resentful and seething. The woman was sharing from the "top table" and in a singsong voice she twittered, "I know I can't, but God Can". I judged her to be a sanctimonious, religion-preaching, idiot, and wanted to slap her. I swore I would never do anything that she suggested.

Time passed and life got tougher. My problems pressed in upon me and I felt like I was drowning. I sat on the end of the bed, fearful and unable to face life. I had thought my rock bottom had been the worst I could feel, but I was wrong. I looked up at the ceiling and said, "Who can help me?" and the thought was immediate, "God Can". I don't go to church, I don't believe in any conventional religion, but I know that when I can't….

It is easy to reject this as a strange idea until we fully understood what it achieves. A God Can is a can or a box that we use to hand over a problem. The activity of making the God Can is an exercise in humility in itself. Put a big label on it – GOD CAN. By writing what the problem is on a piece of paper, we are forcing ourselves to accept that we cannot handle the situation. Once the letter has been "posted", it is no longer ours to worry about. After a time we can go back and have a look at some of the things that were causing us problems, many of them will be long gone and forgotten about. Others did happen, but weren't as frightening as we had expected.

Start a meeting

Starting a new meeting is a great experience and if sobriety seems flat, it is often worth considering setting one up. The involvement it requires is not great, but it destroys complacency.

Everybody involved in a start-up is usually eager to take on any task, from putting out the chairs through to secretarial functions. Most meetings start quite small and this allows time for the people involved to get to know each other. They often allow themselves to share in more depth than they were doing at other meetings. As the meeting expands, these people become the "core" members of the group. It grows and quickly develops a personality. We can watch as our "child" takes its place in the world. There is a pleasant satisfaction in knowing that the group we helped to set up will continue to flourish and help people to find sobriety.

Situations

Situations and Facts

A saying around AA is that our Higher Power won't give us more to cope with than we can handle, many silently add the word "barely". Alcoholism doesn't grant a pardon from the realities of life. Our loved ones sometimes get sick or die and circumstances that we want to go in our favour sometimes don't. Life in the real world means that we encounter real life problems and it can be disturbing.

A living problem can be either a situation or a fact. A situation is a "storm at sea", sometimes the correct action is to batten down the hatches and allow it to wash over us. Once it has passed, we can evaluate the damage and attempt to return to normal. A fact is more like finding that we have to live under the sea. There is no point complaining, no matter how often we try, we can't stroll outside without an oxygen tank. We survive by accepting changes.

Whether we are dealing with a situation or a fact, identifying the nature of the problem allows us to decide on how we can move from "living in the problem," through to "living in the solution". This is one of those glib phrases thrown at us when we feel like we are struggling to keep our head above water. It is easy to see that we are living in the problem, but it takes acceptance, planning and action to achieve living in the solution.

My wife's mother became ill and needed support. The ringing of a telephone snatched time from us that we planned to have together. Strain affected every waking moment. She was certainly dying, but we had no idea if this would be over a period of weeks or years.

I confess to taking a long time to adjust from petulant sulking into being able to support my wife and I needed the support of friends who knew when to listen and when to push. One day it finally clicked, I had to change my role in the home. By taking more responsibility for cooking and shopping, I took some of the pressure off my wife. As I moved towards contributing, I felt useful and my wife gained the freedom to lean on me without fearing the backlash of a childish tantrum. From then on, we could live in the solution, it wasn't an easy time, but I know that we came through it a closer and stronger couple.

Be aware of our role

Although we sometimes upset other people, our new way of life should prove less damaging to those around us. Becoming a sober member of society means people recognise us as reliable. Through humility, we accept that we are not the centre of the universe, other people have rights and responsibilities and things go wrong that are nothing to do with us.

Allow somebody else to have a bad day. We can take it as rejection when somebody seems upset and preoccupied. We don't know if we are the cause of their problems, but we immediately assume that we are. Uncertain of what we have done wrong we either work harder on making them like us, or react badly towards them.

Learning to say no appropriately can be challenging to us. People are usually asking us to do something, give something, or go somewhere. If we decide not to go to a party, we think that people will want to know why we are not there, or if we attend, but leave early, they will want to know why we are leaving. They will rarely miss us as much as we imagine and if we feel that we are putting ourselves at risk - we should not attend.

It can be hard for us to accept that saying yes and helping

somebody can be damaging for them. In the case of somebody who constantly demands support, possibly the best thing we can do for them is to make them sort out their own problems and learn how to cope.

Our confusion can often be a veiled encounter with either high or low self-esteem. "They are asking me because I am the only person who can help," is a sure sign of high self-esteem, whereas fear of rejection in thoughts like "if I say no, they won't forgive me for letting them down" highlights a low self-esteem. They are asking us to put aside what we feel is important in favour of what is important to them. Accepting that we are human is displaying humility and we should not be afraid of saying "no" when we have used sober thinking to decide that it is the correct answer.

Relationships

We might claim to be "experts" at relationships, because we have had hundreds of them. When we look at this honestly, we often have to admit that we are emotionally immature and have a child-like understanding of what a relationship should be. Unrealistically, we imagine the passion of the first days of a love affair will last forever. Amidst the whirlwind of infatuation, we can pass off our immature intensity as love, but relationships change, some fail and others deepen. We sometimes misinterpret a maturing relationship as a failing one and give up on it. We need to learn how to exist successfully within a loving relationship. Discovering, and accepting this frees us to experience the true magic of love, but is possibly one of the most difficult changes we undergo.

Relationships are hard and require willingness to compromise on fundamental aspects of our life. Like recovery from alcoholism, the challenge is that we should be *willing to go to any lengths* to make it work. No matter how hard we try, we cannot make a bad relationship good and we have to acquire the wisdom to understand the dynamics of our situation. The key word is trust, if the relationship is honest and viable, we can have the confidence that our partner will not deliberately harm us, allowing us the freedom to "go to any lengths". Our problem is that we either trust too quickly, or in spite of reassuring evidence, remain reticent. Trust is a decision. More than at any other time, we need to be honest and willing to learn from our past mistakes.

Things other than drinking problems render people incapable of a genuine relationship. The problems are numerous, but for simplicity, it is possible to describe their behaviour as ranging from predator through to victim.

These people don't wear a uniform or carry a badge to identify them and not all predators are male and all victims female. Viewed from the outside the behaviour of both ends of the spectrum seems similar. They progress through relationships in the belief they are looking for "love". The differences are subtle and lie in how they attract their partners and in whom the apparent damage occurs. The predator seems to escape unscathed, leaving an injured partner, whilst the victim appears to receive all of the harm. This isn't true.

I look at my past behaviour and cannot recognise the person who behaved that way. I had no boundaries. I needed love and my need allowed me to justify all of my actions. The wife sitting at home waiting for her husband didn't exist. If I thought of her at all, it was in a disparaging way, if she couldn't satisfy her man then he was bound to stray. I lived without guilt or compassion, statements like, "we are both adults", "he can make his own decisions", defended my right to continue.

I think I frequently had reality upside down. I thought dating a

procession of married men was evidence of my feminine
superiority, proof that no man could resist my deadly beauty. I
now see that they were using me, stroking their ego, allowing
them to boast at how they had hung me upon their arm.

If I failed to dictate the break-up, I always ended up being hurt. I
justified it, hid the anguish and swore "never again". I moved
through relationships like a blind prospector. I went through the
motions of panning, but never found gold.

AA Relationships

Some of the romantic relationships formed within AA turn
out to be good, but many don't. Nobody is naive enough
to embark knowingly on a damaging relationship. It is
only with hindsight that we can see that we ignored the
truth and allowed our desires to overrule our brain.

Whilst people will recognise that they used to be a
predator, they will rarely acknowledge that they still are.
To do so is an admission that we are unwilling to address
our defects. People who are serial victims can also be
alcoholics. The program addresses their alcoholism, not
their other issues. Until they gain the confidence to look
for ways to tackle them, they will remain in danger. The
victim's apparent inability to identify predators means
that they will almost certainly attract unhealthy attention
within the rooms. When the relationship turns sour, the
victim usually develops a strong resentment. They
complain that the people at the meeting should have
protected them. They feel betrayed and turn their back on
the meeting forgetting why they came in the first place.

"T" was an attractive girl who laughingly confessed that her
answer to any problem was to find a man to help her. Although
many of the women tried to talk to her, she ignored their advice.
She would visit the meetings, attract men with as little sobriety
as she had and then vanish for months. Her looks faded as she

took a series of emotional and physical beatings. She told of waking up in a graveyard with a black eye and a missing tooth, but still sought salvation through a relationship. She became pregnant and had a child damaged by pre-natal alcohol syndrome. She abandoned her daughter when she hit the streets for the last time – still searching for the man who would save her.

Not all AA relationships are of a predatory / victim nature. They can occur between two consenting adults and still prove to be damaging and result in one or both of them drinking. The claim that an affair "just happened" is a fiction from storybooks. An affair requires two factors *Urge* and *Opportunity*. Either can occur spontaneously, but for them to coincide requires planning. Having decided to embark upon a path of lies and deceit, we should not expect our sobriety to survive.

Even when both parties are free, alcoholism adds an extra dimension of complexity. We are constantly in a state of recovery or relapse. When arguments occur, our knowledge of the program provides a ready supply of barbed weapons for us to throw. Sniping shots such as, "go and see your sponsor", or "you're not on the program", might be accurate, but they are usually inappropriate between partners. People in successful AA relationships say that it is essential to keep recovery separate. They respect each other's need to attend their own chosen meetings. When they discuss recovery, they discuss it the same way as an alcoholic and non-alcoholic would, resisting any temptation towards "tough love sponsorship", but offering loving support.

Non-AA Relationships

Although we possibly arrived in AA with a partner, it is rare for such a relationship to survive unchanged. Our partner will be responding to the person they knew, but recovery changes us more than they anticipate. Our love affair often needs to start afresh and allow both partners to discover who the other really is. When this occurs, our relationship doesn't usually just survive, but flourishes. The suggestion that we don't make any major decisions in the first two years of recovery has preserved many marriages, but just as in the rest of society, some fail and some succeed.

We can emerge into recovery having lost, or having never had a partner, but it is quite normal to hope to find a stable relationship. The partner from within AA comes with a guarantee of instability. Outside it remains a lottery. There is more sickness in the world than alcoholism and the more sinister forms can be hard to identify. If we feel that everybody we get involved with is unstable, we possibly ought to look at the common factor – us. The new love of our life could start out as the most stable person we had ever met, but become worn down by our intensity. We can be unpredictable, dependent and jealous and many people are not willing to tolerate this. We have to be willing to accept their criticism and decide if we want to make the effort to change.

We all have rights. We have the right to go to meetings and to continue to grow. They have the right to continue to go into drinking situations and pursue their life without carrying the burden of our alcoholism.

Drinking Situations

We can't have a social life based in the tavern, but we can attend the special occasions that occur. Although alcohol will be present, it isn't the main reason for the function. These events are important to the people we care about and they will expect us to attend. Recovery means that we are able to go without drinking or feeling threatened. To do so successfully, it is vital to adopt a protective attitude and remain vigilant when we are around alcohol. The thought of a drink can seem distant, but once the monkey is aroused, it moves up a gear in the attempt to take control. The best advice is never to go into a situation where drink is available without taking a quick check on our sobriety, using questions like:

- "Should I be going?"

- "Why am I going?"

- "Am I irrationally bad tempered before going?"

- "Do I feel the need to prove a point here?"

If we have doubt about any of these points or feel uncertain for some reason then we would be far safer to decide that it is foolish to go. Emotion runs high at weddings, christenings and funerals. Parties and gatherings of old friends can unexpectedly throw up resentment, jealousy and anger, providing the monkey with a vast array of insidious thoughts to use. These thoughts can come upon us at any time, but when they occur and there is drink available, we have a serious problem. We should always take steps to protect ourselves, such as making sure that there isn't a wine glass positioned close to our hand. Many of us have been surprised to find our glasses switched whilst we weren't looking, waiters and other guests are not responsible for our drink – we are.

We can usually spot the people who will become drunk as the party progresses. In the past, we would have been part of or even the centre of this group, but it is much safer to stay away. Until we have adjusted our thinking to recognise that this group is not the "real" party they are a threat. They will drag us into enthusiastic reflection on past exploits. We might possibly gaze upon them with contempt, seeing them as "amateur" drinkers and want to show them how to do it properly. Amongst this group is the person who resents or is contemptuous of our efforts to remain sober and they are capable of deliberately swapping our glass.

By anticipating the situations and feelings we may encounter, we can enjoy rather than endure the party. If we feel uneasy, there is no substitute for speaking to another sober alcoholic and carrying a few contact numbers can save our life. Failing this, we should always have an "escape route" planned and the humility to use it.

Dinner with friends

When ordering drinks from a waiter, it is a good idea to order last. It is then easy to choose a drink that looks different from the rest of the order. If the rest of the party is having gin and tonic, we can order a cola rather than a tonic. Thoughts like *why should I be the one to change*, or *I want tonic water* occasionally arise, but learning to think defensively around drink is an exercise in humility and a small price to pay to enjoy the rest of the evening. Why have little bits of stress we don't need?

Avoid - handling drink

For many years after I got sober, I happily handled drinks. I would go to the bar and serve wine at the dinner table. If we had visitors, we would open a bottle of wine and leave it in the kitchen. I would act as host, refilling glasses as required. One evening I stood in the kitchen pouring a glass of wine and the thought "taste it" hit me like a brick on a rope. The voice suggesting that, "nobody will know" was almost irresistibly.

The urge to take a drink was overwhelming and frightening.

Of course, I didn't mention this feeling to anybody, not wishing to make a fuss "at my time in sobriety". Within the week I sat at a meeting listening to somebody recount how with seven years sobriety, he had done exactly what I had considered. For him, it had meant a couple of years of secret drinking and a downward spiral before achieving a second rock bottom.

If possible, it is sensible to avoid handling drink. We are not "being a wimp", but exhibiting humility by recognising that there are things we should not do. If we have to handle bottles, a useful suggestion is to imagine that we can see a bright red skull and cross bones with the word, POISON printed on the label. Whilst suggestions like this can seem childish, we should use any trick that works.

Avoid - Booze in food

When we obviously avoid a dish with alcohol in it, it is surprising how often people feel obliged to explain that cooking burns it off. The person might be somebody influential and important to our lives, creating an unexpected dilemma. Do we have the strength of character to stick with our conviction? In doing so, we are effectively saying they are wrong and risking offending them.

If we choose to order food with alcohol, we create an opening for the monkey. The illness can point out how we "got away with it" and how much better the dish had tasted, but it also opens other dangers. Amongst the people at the table, we are no longer a person who doesn't have alcohol. Now, without a firm line drawn, they will feel obliged to offer a small glass of wine or liqueur with the meal. These friends may have always felt we were slightly "cranky" in our decision to give up drinking and hoping that our resolve has weakened, may try to help us get over our silly obsession.

Our partner is sitting close by, is possibly seeing the doorway to hell open up before them. In silent anguish, they wonder if this is the start of a slide back into full-blown alcoholic behaviour. Under these circumstances, they might not be the sparkling companion we had expected, detecting their coldness, we react badly and escalate the situation into an argument.

All we did was simply choose a dish off the menu, just like any other person in the restaurant. Why should we feel guilty about that? We all know that science says that alcohol burns off during cooking, but few are educated to the level required to explain the atomic structure of the alcohol. Nobody has yet identified the part of the molecule that triggers the illness, or proved that heat destroys this specific part of the atomic combination. If it is destroyed, how long does it take and at what temperature?

These are the complicated and pseudo-scientific arguments. The simple fact is that an alcoholic should avoid knowingly consuming alcohol. If we start to justify it, what is the next step in our thinking?

Christmas

There is a joke about a turkey that was all excited and looking forward to Christmas and the irony of it applies equally well to an alcoholic. It is natural to want to enjoy ourselves and we can, on condition that we monitor our feelings and are prepared to take rapid action to address them.

This is one of the most emotionally charged times of the

year and people feel they deserve a good time. Corporations spend huge advertising budgets to convince us that if we drink their brand of alcohol, we will join a happy party world of log fires and elegant people laughing in merry delight. If the only place our drinking had taken us had been amongst people with perfect smiles, drinking from delicate glasses – we wouldn't have a problem.

At any meeting, a "wise sage" will explain that there are 24 hours in Christmas day and we live through them the same way as we do any other day. This is true, but whilst this single day is the focus, the holiday of Christmas extends to several days and planning how to get through each of these "extra stressful" 24-hour days is essential.

It can be easy for us to become so busy with the festivities that we feel unable to attend our regular meetings. If it seems laughable when somebody suggests that we should be attending extra ones, it is time to stop and review reality. *We are busy because of sobriety, not in spite of it* and missing meetings because they are inconvenient is complacency. Regardless of how well we are feeling there are reasons why we should try to attend more meetings than normal.

<u>Working our twelfth step</u>, we will almost certainly meet people who are not enjoying the holiday. Our first Christmas is usually difficult to live through. It is a time when morbid reflection on our past can become attractive. In this mood, we magnify the virtue of what we lost and the stupidity of how we lost it. Being amongst other people who have passed through similar darkness into a happy way of life is vital to help us survive.

<u>Recognising our own stress levels</u>, we are likely to find that the meeting highlights how we have been running at

a higher stress level than we normally do and brings us back down to earth. Meetings leave us better equipped to take part in the festivities. By allowing ourselves the time to go to them, we are not selfishly spoiling Christmas for the rest of our family, but trying to ensure that we don't spoil it.

If we attend meetings and make sure we keep in touch with other alcoholics, we can enjoy ourselves. As we progress, there is always one Christmas that gives us a lot of trouble and so even though we handled the last one without a problem we should not drift into the coming one without fully preparing ourselves.

Holidays

For most people, their holiday is the most expensive regular purchase they make and it is easy to expect too much from it. Our emotions simmer and we cry "why me, why now!" as we hear news of disruption on the roads or airlines. The monkey brings them to the boil when it disrupts our thinking with ideas like, "I deserve to be treated better than this", or "all I want is two weeks relaxation". We think that we are alone in our feelings, but more people experience stress related headaches and back pain during their holiday than at any other time of the year. Providing we plan appropriately, they are an opportunity to relax and unwind, but they are not worth risking our sobriety over.

Can we afford it? Companies design holiday brochures to tempt us into spending more than we can afford. We can justify to ourselves that we deserve the holiday, but if we are creating stress by spending too much money, we will almost certainly experience a backlash from it when we get home.

<u>Where are we going?</u> A part of the planning needs to include deciding on the holiday destination. Most of us don't cope well with rowdy drunks and so even if it is a "bargain", certain resorts are probably not a wise choice.

If we are attracted to a rowdy resort, we should check our motives. The lure of toned bodies and balmy nights can seem extremely appealing, especially if this coincides with our recovery feeling a little flat. Are we really planning to have a relaxing time, or are we planning to indulge ourselves, claiming that the atmosphere of the place overwhelmed us? The plan may not include drinking, but it can often result in it.

<u>Who will go with us?</u> We need to be amongst people we can trust to support us if we need them to. It is often wrong for us to plan to be on our own. It is also wrong to go with somebody who is resentful or ignorant of our alcoholism. We don't need the stress created by worrying that somebody could "treat us" to a shot of booze in our soft drink.

<u>How are we going to stay sober?</u> We need to think about this before we travel rather than realise that we are in danger when we get there. Whether we use it or not, it is always worth spending the time to get the local AA telephone number and find out when and where the meetings will be. Few holiday destinations are "hundreds of miles" from AA and a visit to the local meeting can be part of the holiday. Obviously, it is more difficult as a single parent with young children, but we should not travel without a plan.

It is sensible to take some AA literature to read. The beach is a great place to read up on the steps and traditions and if we feel self-conscious, we can always put it into the cover from another book. It is not difficult to stay in touch with people by telephone and spending part of our old drinking budget on calls would allow most of us to plan a daily chat with an AA friend from home.

Moving House

We sometimes have to move away from the area where we originally got sober. We know that it is not difficult to find a meeting anywhere in the world, but whilst visiting a new meeting is often worthwhile, they are rarely as fulfilling as our home group.

I have moved area twice during my sobriety. The first time was a temporary re-location about sixty miles north of my home group. I found that the local meetings were not what I expected and I preferred to have a long drive back to enjoy a "real" meeting rather than to try to fit in locally. This was difficult when the winter came and I missed quite a few meetings because of bad weather, but I soon returned home and settled back into my comfortable meetings.

I changed my job and the new company asked me to move much further North. This time, I knew that it was too far and that I had to settle in to the local meetings. The first one seemed like a bunch of misfits trying to avoid reality and the second was full of people twittering about serenity and prayer. I think of myself as down to earth and I want meetings that talk about the twelve steps and drinking. I judged all of the local meetings based upon my first two and decided that I would attend as few of them as possible and try self-sponsorship.

My new employer fell into difficulties, made me redundant and I suddenly found myself in emotional free fall. I knew that I had to either change or drink. I decided to attempt ninety meetings in ninety days to re-engage myself with AA. With this new burst of activity, I found some groups that I enjoyed and people to support me. A new sponsor emerged and I survived what I can see was an extremely dangerous time.

When a new face appears at a meeting, they are usually warmly welcomed and it is easy to fall into a trap of "assumed" sobriety. The people at the meeting may be deceived into believing that we are coping and our pride won't let us confess to these strangers that we need help.

Regardless of length of sobriety, we will immediately benefit from throwing ourselves into meetings and getting to know as many local alcoholics as possible. By doing this, we quickly establish a good support network. We should also make a conscious effort to find a new sponsor and identify people that we can talk to on a one to one basis.

When we make this renewed effort, we often see that we had fallen into a rut at our old meetings, that we were guilty of attending in body, but not in mind. Our move becomes a positive re-introduction into sobriety and we start to grow again.

Removing Resentment

Our toughest obstacle can be removing a strongly held resentment against another person. The Big Book contains a method guaranteed to work. However, when we first encounter it, we almost certainly recoil with horror at the suggestion. It works and thousands of us have improved our lives by using it.

My wife had left me for a mutual friend and I was devastated. I wanted both of them to die a miserable, slow, painful death and the thought of them enjoying life constantly gnawed at my thoughts. My sponsor suggested praying for them to have everything I would wish for myself. I thought he was joking and I emphatically refused to contemplate it. The suffering continued, but my sponsor wouldn't offer any other solution, he simply repeated the suggestion. I finally gave in and tried it. Every day for two weeks, twice a day (and sometimes more frequently), I prayed for them. I didn't notice when I changed from belligerently following instructions into meaning it, but it happened. I then realised that I felt better, my repetitive fixation vanished and my life blossomed.

The Big Book explains that we are not doing this for their benefit, but for us. We are the beneficiaries of this activity and so to hold back from it is to remain in pain pointlessly. The willingness to try to succeed with this exercise shows that we have finally started to grow into a spiritual way of living beyond anything we could have conceived for ourselves.

Printed in Great
Britain
by Amazon